DEATH OF A DREAM

BY DONNA HOHMANN EWY AND RODGER FRANK EWY

Preparation for Childbirth

Preparation for Breastfeeding

The Cycle of Life:
Guide to a Healthy Pregnancy
Guide to Family-Centered Childbirth
Guide to Parenting: You and Your Newborn

Teen Pregnancy: Challenges and Choices

Miscarriage, Stillbirth, and Newborn Loss

DEATH OF A DREAM

Donna Hohmann Ewy and Rodger Frank Ewy

Foreword by Marshall Klaus, M.D.

E. P. DUTTON, INC. • NEW YORK

Published in the United States by E. P. Dutton, Inc.,
2 Park Avenue, New York, N.Y. 10016

Library of Congress Cataloging in Publication Data
Ewy, Donna.
Death of a dream.

Bibliography: p.
1. Miscarriage. 2. Still-birth. 3. Infants (Newborn)
—Mortality. 4. Children—Death—Psychological aspects.
5. Parents—Psychology. I. Ewy, Rodger. II. Title.
RG648.E95 1984 155.9'37 84-1465

ISBN: 0-525-48080-3

Published simultaneously in Canada by
Fitzhenry & Whiteside Limited, Toronto

W

Designed by Mark O'Connor

10 9 8 7 6 5 4 3 2 1

First Edition

Dedicated to

Elizabeth
Elyssa
Christian
Stephan
Juliana

Written by, with and for
The Boulder County Hospice Stillborn/
Newborn Loss Support Group
and Other Bereaved Parents

Our greatest appreciation to all the parents who shared their experiences, their sadness, and their joys with us to make this book possible. With special thanks to: Martha and Leslie Anderson, Rosalyn and Peter Berntsen, Nicki and Scott Canby, Nancy and Bob Rands, Virginia and James Trinidad, and to Marcia Lattanzi who made all this possible.

We wish to thank Ted Appel, M.D., and Edward Brown, M.D., who generously shared their time with us in hopes of helping other medical staff personnel better fulfill the needs of bereaved parents. Boulder Community Hospital and its staff opened its doors to us. Leon Ewy spent hours reading, editing, and typing. Nancy Rands not only shared herself in a parenting capacity but also as an editor. And finally, Karen Braziller, our editor at Dutton, gave the support, patience, and encouragement, without which this book would not have been completed.

Contents

Foreword

In times past, the procedures following the death of an infant were managed within the family. The body of the dead infant was viewed in the home, and the family, with continuing community support, actively participated in the funeral. Today, however, the hospital has often taken over the process of both an infant's entering and leaving conscious existence. Customs and traditions, developed over many hundreds of years to aid the normal course of grieving and mourning for survivors, have in part been lost, and many in our society are unfamiliar with how to help parents who lose a newborn. With unusual sensitivity the authors bring insight, understanding, and useful information to parents who have experienced such losses and to those professionals and others who are in the position of helping parents through such times.

Although each parent tends to go through a similar series of reactions including shock, disbelief, anger, sadness, loss of normal relationships and patterns of activity, it is necessary for parents to understand that each individual may go through the process at a different rate, stopping at some stages for longer or shorter periods of time. It's not uncommon that because of the asynchronous movement through the process of grieving, parents can become estranged from each other. Therefore, it is especially helpful for parents to remember to check with each other at some time each day to see how the other is managing.

The death of a newborn or a stillbirth is a crisis for any couple. Parents can help each other by listening and talking to one another, being patient with and caring for each other, touching each other, and if need be, by crying together and accepting each other's intense sadness. Without mutual listening and understanding, one or both of the partners, either the father or the mother, may not adequately grieve the loss.

The authors carefully describe these difficult feelings, thoughts, and ideas, sometimes using the real words of parents going through their painful times. As one mother noted, "The loss of the baby is, in part, a loss of part of yourself that can almost never be made up." Another parent feels her baby still moving inside. A father learns about his wife's true thoughts at a group meeting. The normal parents in this book talk movingly about a major event in their lives.

The many recommendations in this book are strongly supported by clinical observations and emphasize that it is most helpful for the father and mother's future normal life that they fully experience the pain and sadness and true loss that has occurred. When medically feasible, parents can hold the baby while it is dying. They should have time with their infant in the hospital after the death, or, if the baby is stillborn they should have time to see and hold the baby.

In parent groups where families discuss and share their feelings with others who have lost an infant, they often talk about how much they missed not having time with the baby after the death. Ten or twenty years ago the practice of most hospitals was to remove the baby quickly and suggest to the parents that they get back to their usual course of living. It is now clear that this can lead to long-term problems for one or both parents. It is necessary that they go through the process of grieving described in this book. Thus friends and relatives, physicians and nurses, are especially helpful when they are able to listen to the sadness, anger, and hostility, as well as to some of the crazy and mixed-up thoughts that normal parents have during the agonizing period after an infant's death.

I have learned much from listening to parents during group meetings. In these meetings parents have mentioned distressing thoughts such as concern about going crazy or the urge to commit suicide; however, they frequently note that hearing about the experiences of other parents gives them the courage to carry on. Almost invariably there is criticism of physicians and nurses. It is important to listen to these thoughts and impressions and not to defend the care or caretakers, even when the criticism is so directed. In almost every group meeting parents express their great concern that others will forget about the baby. They experience a need to make a strong effort to have others remember. "You want to shout to the world that your baby has lived and you don't want the world to forget." They all agree about the terrible pain, the severe feelings of emptiness, and that no one can appreciate the pain and misery except someone who has also lost an infant.

Group meetings are not for all parents. Each individual has different ways of approaching and managing experience; however, as a principle it is important not to suppress one's thoughts or feelings. The majority of parents agree that the most helpful ingredients for moving through grief and restoring the self are those friends, relatives, and caretakers who are able to listen sympathetically and quietly to their sad and upsetting thoughts. After observing adverse effects for many years, most professionals believe it is important to wait before starting another pregnancy until one has finished grieving the infant who died. It is necessary to give up one baby before parents can attach to or develop a tie to the new infant. Otherwise, the two infants can become merged, in a complex fashion, in the parents' minds.

When the grief process does not proceed normally, pathological grief can ensue. Symptoms include: (1) Overactivity without a sense of loss; (2) adoption of the symptoms belonging to the last illness of the deceased (in the case of loss of a close adult); (3) the onset of new diseases such as ulcerative colitis, asthma, or rheumatoid arthritis; (4) severe alterations in relationships with friends or relatives; (5) furious hostility against a specific person; (6) lasting loss of patterns of social interaction; (7) actions detrimental to one's own social or economic existence; as well as (8) agitated depression. Such parents will need additional guidance from skilled psychiatric personnel to pass safely through this difficult period of their lives.

This caring, poignant, and well-documented book written for both parents and professionals describes in detail the many important stages, issues, and variations of the grief experience surrounding fetal or neonatal loss. In addition, the authors have denoted clear and helpful suggestions for constructive actions and coping during this period and for eventually moving forward.

—MARSHALL KLAUS, M.D., CHAIRMAN
DEPARTMENT OF PEDIATRICS/HUMAN DEVELOPMENT,
MICHIGAN STATE UNIVERSITY

Preface

From the moment of conception, whether the pregnancy was planned or not, all parents begin to wonder what their baby will bring to their lives; they begin to dream dreams of the future. While all parents have concerns over the possibility of something going wrong, few childbirth educators or physicians acknowledge, even to themselves, the potential for stillbirth or newborn death. When a pregnancy ends in death, every parent grieves the death of a dream. We hope this book shows the impact of the death on parents, and on the health care professionals involved.

For every 3.3 million live births in the United States, national health statistics show that 800,000 parents lose their babies from miscarriage, 30,000 lose their babies to stillbirth, and 33,000 babies die shortly after birth. No parent is prepared for such a tragedy.

Acknowledging the right of the parents to grieve and providing support are the most significant elements in helping parents deal with their loss. Mothers and fathers have distinct differences in their responses to loss and in their grieving. As a group, mothers feel more bonded to the child and feel more strongly that the child was a "real person." Fathers often feel left out of that aspect, and they also receive less support. The differences in the grieving styles can significantly affect the marriage. Subsequent pregnancies do not "make up for" or replace the child who died. The experience of a miscarriage, stillbirth, or neonatal death is one that parents find changes their lives forever. How their needs are met by staff, family, and friends will affect how they cope with their grief.

Death of a Dream explores the experiences of parents who have lost their babies. Few doctors, nurses, childbirth educators, friends, or family members know how to help ease the pain these parents suffer. This book also deals with methods that most help parents in the hours, days, and months following their loss.

The results of hours of interviews with parents, doctors, nurses, friends, and support staff have been compiled in this guide for parents whose babies have died, whether in miscarriage, stillbirth, or shortly after birth. The first part of the book focuses on the reasons for fetal and neonatal death, and the hospital stay and what it entails. The middle section is a discussion of grief, both immediate and long-term, including suggestions on how the parents can help each other work their way through grief and how their family and friends can help them. The third part addresses itself to the future, to subsequent pregnancies, and, for most parents, healthy births.

DEATH OF A DREAM

Daniel Brubacher
(direct translation from the German)

Family Register of Daniel Brubacher. 1844

May 27, 1844	—We were married and have to remain so until God does us part.
December 7, 1845	—God gave us a daughter Maria. She died April 28, 1847.
April 23, 1847	—God gave us a son, Heinrich.
November 19, 1848	—God gave us a son, Johann. He died January 15, 1849.
January 18, 1850	—God gave us a daughter, Maria.
January 9, 1852	—A daughter was born to us. She died January 11, 1852.
May 13, 1853	—A daughter, Katherina, was born to us. She died June 4, 1854.
April 8, 1855	—A son, Johann, was born to us.
June 24, 1857	—A daughter, Elisabeth, was born to us. She died March 3, 1858.
May 15, 1859	—A daughter which we named Barbara was born to us.
May 27, 1861	—A daughter, Elisabeth, was born to us.
August 20, 1863	—A son, Peter, was born to us.
April 23, 1864	—God gave us another son, Jakob.
June 17, 1864	—Our daughter Maria died after a long illness.
July 6, 1868	—Another daughter was born to us, against all expectations. We gave her the name Christine.

A Lesson from History

While working on this book I discovered the page facing this one in the family Bible of Daniel Brubacher, Rodger's great-grandfather. In its stark simplicity it emphasized only too clearly that babies have always died. Out of fourteen babies born only six children survived, and any miscarriages between births were not even mentioned.

Miscarriage, stillbirth, and newborn death have always been—and will always be—with us. It is only in the last few decades in a world of increasing scientific and medical technology that parents have been given to expect that if the mother follows good nutritional guidelines, gets early prenatal care, and "takes good care of herself," they are assured a healthy baby. Unfortunately, this expectation is unrealistic, and the harmful implication is that if the baby dies, the mother did something wrong. Thus parents who have lost a baby have felt an overwhelming burden of guilt and failure and sometimes see themselves as "freaks of nature."

For parents whose babies have died, the feelings of guilt and failure can be replaced with an understanding that, through no fault of their own, these things do happen in life. We must somehow prepare each generation for the predictable unpredictability that has always been a part of life. Death, illness, and pain are all normal parts of life that each of us will have to face at some time. It is not a question of *if* but *when* and *how* they must be faced.

I

Attachment and Loss

1

The Dream

Although the parents interviewed in this book were of different ages and backgrounds they all shared in the excitement of pregnancy and loved their babies as cherished members of their families. These parents expected normal, healthy births, but instead lost their babies to death. Some experienced miscarriages, some stillbirths, and some saw their critically ill babies linger briefly and die. Each was totally unprepared for the death.

Not only were these parents unprepared, but they found that almost all doctors, nurses, family members, and friends who surrounded them during the death were equally unprepared. It was not that they didn't want to help the parents, but most of them simply did not know how. Those who had a special understanding, knowledge, and skill were able to provide comfort that supported parents in their grief and allowed them to work through their sorrow.

Part of the tragedy is that parents are led to believe that if the mother eats a nutritious diet, receives good prenatal care, and delivers at a hospital, a live, healthy baby will be born. When expectant parents express to the doctors the normal fears that all experience: "What if my baby is not normal?", "What if my baby dies?", doctors assure them that 97–98 percent of all pregnancies end in a normal, healthy birth, and that the parents are "not to worry." Thus parents who lose their babies feel like freaks or failures. Today, no one—not parent, family, friends, doctor, or medical staff—expects a baby to die or is even prepared to give the parents the comfort and support that is needed.

All parents who have experienced the death of a baby need:

1. Reassurance that they did the best possible job;
2. Support from family, friends, and medical staff;
3. Information as to why this happened;
4. Permission to grieve;
5. Affirmation that the baby had been born and had died;
6. The opportunity to make choices that would affect the parents both in the present and the future.

When the staff, family, and friends help grieving parents fill these needs, they give them the strength needed to cope with the tragedy of a baby's death.

BEFORE CONCEPTION

Recent research shows that parents start to love their children long before they ever conceive. Only when family, friends, and staff are able to see the depth of this love can they begin to give the support needed after the loss of a baby.

> "Our doctor acted like we had just lost a thing. He couldn't even begin to imagine that we had lost our child whom we had loved and cherished for sixteen weeks."

From the time people realize that someday they may be parents, they begin to envision how they will parent and the kind of children they will bring into this world. They think about all the things their own parents did that they do not want to do to their children, and the things their parents did that they want to continue and pass on to their own families. As men and women enter into courtship, they may talk about these dreams and sort through their relationships, centering in on the type of person they would like to parent their future children. Already they are beginning to protect the future of their children.

CONCEPTION

Conception is to many parents a realization of the tremendous role they play in the whole past, present, and future of mankind. Conception means that they will pass on their heritage to the next generation. It means that they will fulfill their reproductive hopes. It means that together they have created a product of their love. Because of all this, they develop great feelings of attachment toward the baby.

FIRST TRIMESTER

THE MOTHER

When a woman first realizes she is pregnant, her joy with the creation of life is mixed with concerns. She has fears of miscarriage, and may even have disturbing dreams about birth and death. As she becomes concerned about her baby's health and accepts her pregnancy as a reality, she begins her first important step in her transition to the role of being a mother.

> "I had been trying to get pregnant for several years. I had lived for conception. When the pregnancy was first confirmed I just couldn't believe it. Then I was wild

> with joy. I knew it was too early—but I couldn't help myself—I ran out and told the world—and my husband ran out and bought the biggest teddy bear he could find. We started making plans for a nursery right away."

THE FATHER

During this time the father may experience ambivalent feelings about the role of fatherhood. A young father may often feel trapped by the new sense of responsibility. He may have trouble relating to the baby at this stage and may actually be disturbed that his wife is so preoccupied with something that he has no or few feelings about.

> "I hate to admit it but even though I tried to act excited, it was hard for me to believe that there was really a baby there. I knew intellectually that my wife was pregnant, but emotionally I think I really hadn't accepted the fact."

SECOND TRIMESTER

THE MOTHER

During the second trimester the mother's first awareness of her baby's movements are accompanied by feelings of wonder and delight. She becomes more and more preoccupied with her baby and herself. She begins to perceive the baby as part of herself, while at the same time she recognizes that the baby is a separate individual. Feeling the fluttering movements causes her to begin fantasizing what her baby will be like. She begins to give him or her a personality. She may purchase clothes, pick out names, and arrange the home to accommodate her baby. As her baby grows within her, she talks to him or her; she might sing her favorite lullabies and rhythmically stroke her abdomen.

> "It was like a miracle. It started off like the soft fluttering of a butterfly or the soft brushing of eyelashes. It's hard to explain. I didn't say anything at first, but every day it got a little stronger. It was the sweetest feeling I ever had. Our baby was alive and moving within me."

THE FATHER

Once the father begins to feel the baby's movements the baby becomes more real to him. He sees himself in the role of a father. During the second trimester the father may find it difficult to adjust to his wife's fluctuating emotions. Her preoccupation with herself and the baby may leave him feeling neglected and jealous.

> "It was pretty tough. One day she would be so happy and on top of the world. The next, she would be down in the dumps and hard to get along with. I tried to be understanding but sometimes I would just leave the house and go out with my buddies for relief from all that stuff."

THIRD TRIMESTER

THE MOTHER

During the third trimester the mother begins to prepare for the birth of her baby. Extreme mood swings from exuberance to depression are common. She is concerned about her baby's health and her ability to mother. She may begin to take childbirth classes with the father in preparation for a healthy and safe delivery. If she is working, she must rearrange her life to take on the most important job of her life—motherhood. Friends give her baby showers; grandparents anticipate the arrival of the baby; siblings await the new life in their family.

The mother may experience feelings of anxiety about labor and delivery. As her pregnancy nears term, she may have recurring fears and dreams about birth, death, and deformed or retarded children.

> "Toward the end of my pregnancy I must have been a bear to live with. I know that my husband had a hard time putting up with my emotional ups and downs. I couldn't help it. I went from elation to depression and back up again. No one knew what to expect."

> "It was the best part of my pregnancy. I waddled around feeling like 'Mother Earth.' This is what I had always wanted. I read somewhere that you could program your child to like music, so I used to hold a music box against my stomach and played Chopin's 'Polonaise' for hours. I would go around the house humming and singing to my baby. I was absolutely sure that she heard me; I was raising a future piano virtuoso."

THE FATHER

Now the baby is a reality for the father. He may talk to the baby. As he feels the form of his baby through the mother's abdomen, he "sees" the feet, arms, and legs as the baby moves. By now the parents may have picked out a name or have given the baby a nickname. They may spend hours making plans for the baby who will soon be born. They might even think about the baby's future and make plans as far off as college.

Along with the sense of responsibility and plans for financial security, the labor and delivery, and the health of the baby begin to be real concerns. It is not uncommon for men to experience vivid dreams at this time and also to have fears concerning the birth, death, and possible deformity or retardation of the baby.

"My favorite part of the pregnancy was when we would go to bed at night and we would watch our baby move. You could actually see its elbows and knees moving. I know it's hard to believe, but I would lay my hand on my wife's tummy and the baby would quiet down. We called it the 'soothing hand.'"

2

Miscarriage

Out of every 100 conceptions, at least twenty end in miscarriage. Every parent who experiences a miscarriage is totally unprepared for this eventuality. Society had promised a healthy baby, and the parents were not prepared for the unexpected, for the bleeding or the pain, or for the indifference of the doctors' and society's response toward their pain and grief.

Although the babies were not fully developed physically, the expectant parent had already given them personalities and personhoods. When they died, the grief was profound. "Why did our baby die? What happened? What went wrong?" Many times after miscarriage, the mother has deep feelings of guilt. "What did I do to cause this? Is my body at fault?" Many mothers question their ability to conceive and their future as parents.

DEFINITION OF MISCARRIAGE

Miscarriage is the termination of a pregnancy between conception and the 20th week of gestation. Seventy-five percent of all miscarriages take place before the thirteenth week. Miscarriage ends in two ways. Spontaneous abortion is when the baby is expelled through the vagina without any medical intervention. Induced abortion is the interruption of pregnancy and expulsion of the fetus by external medical means.

The exact incidence of miscarriage is not known because statistics do not include those women who miscarried but who did not see a doctor, or who experienced it only as a delayed or unusually heavy menstrual period. However, for those recorded, at least one in five pregnancies ends in miscarriage.

JUDY AND STEVEN

MISCARRIAGE AT 6 WEEKS

Steven and I had been trying for six months to conceive a baby. Although I hadn't told anyone, I was overjoyed when I missed my period. When the doctor confirmed my pregnancy, we were ecstatic and went out to celebrate. About a week later I noticed some blood when I went to the bathroom. I took time off from work and went right to bed, because Steven and I really wanted this baby. I was relieved when my nausea was gone but I began to be suspicious when I noticed that my breasts seemed less full and tender. One night the faint streaks were not faint but bright red. There was a lot, and I began cramping. When the pains became so severe that I couldn't breathe, Steven called the doctor and rushed me to the hospital. Two hours later I delivered what to them was just blood and tissue, but what to me was my baby. The next morning I had a D & C to remove any other tissue that might cause bleeding.

That was the worst experience of my life. I've talked to a lot of my friends and family since then, and I found out that many of them had had the same experience. But they only talk in whispers about it, keeping it in the closet. It's as though they feel guilt for something, as if they are some kind of failures.

CINDY AND ALLEN

MISCARRIAGE AT 16 WEEKS

I had planned the whole pregnancy just as I had planned my life. After completing my degree and working for eight years, my husband and I were ready to start our family. When I stopped using the pill I was surprised when I didn't get pregnant right away. But after eight months of trying I was overjoyed when I had missed my first period. The doctor confirmed my pregnancy and I was ready to proceed with the birth. Although I had had intermittent spotting, it cleared up and when I began to feel my baby moving I was thrilled and sure that everything was okay. After another four weeks, I noticed more bleeding. I contacted my doctor and he told me to get off my feet and see if the bleeding stopped. It did; I went back to work and didn't give much thought to it until several weeks later when I noticed again bright red blood. I was terrified this time and just knew it was something serious. That night I awakened with severe cramping and called my doctor, and again he soothed me and told me to stay in bed. He didn't mention miscarriage. This continued into the next day. That afternoon my water broke and I ran frightened to the bathroom. As I sat on the toilet my baby, so tiny but so well formed, came out in the water. I could see its features, its eyes and little fingers and toes. I nearly fainted.

I called my neighbor and she came over to help me. We called the doctor and he told me he would meet me at the hospital immediately. My husband met us there. He was in shock because he had wanted this baby almost more than I had; it was a real loss to him. Even though I had spotted before, he never wanted to admit that anything might be wrong. Now our worst nightmares had come true. Since I had lost a lot of blood, I felt very faint and as if this was something happening to someone else. It couldn't be me.

After I went home from the hospital and the shock wore off, all I could think of was, "What did I do wrong? Why did my body fail me? Did I wait too long?" I felt like a failure. The doctor said we could have another baby right away, but I really didn't feel like it. I couldn't risk another failure so soon. My husband wanted to try, but we couldn't talk about it. It's been very quiet at our house. Where we expected the presence of a little baby, there is only the shadow of a silent ghost.

What really got to me was that I couldn't talk to anyone about it. Everyone seemed to think that it was just a minor event. No one seemed to understand that I had not only lost my baby that I had loved and carried for almost four months, but I had lost something else in my life.

LOIS AND JOHN

MULTIPLE MISCARRIAGE

John and I married when we were in our mid-twenties and made the decision to start both of our careers before we started our family. When I became pregnant the first time and experienced a miscarriage, the doctor told us not to worry, that it was probably just a freak of nature and we would be able to have more children. I remember being somewhat depressed, but I accepted his word. Nine months later I became pregnant again and early in the pregnancy I was terrified when I started bleeding and cramping, the same way I had in the first pregnancy. This second loss was much more serious because we didn't just lose our baby—I was beginning to doubt my ability to have a baby.

I was extremely hesitant to try again because I just wasn't up to another failure, but my husband was really eager to try. I guess I also felt that I wasn't getting any younger and that my "biological time clock" wasn't going to give me the luxury of waiting around.

The third miscarriage was devastating to both John and me. I was panicked and terrified. This meant not only the death of our baby, but maybe the death of our hopes of having a family. I went into a deep depression.

Although I had felt success before in my career, I now felt only failure. My self-esteem, my self-confidence were gone; I wasn't even interested in how I looked or how the house looked. I couldn't seem to get the energy to get on with my life.

Finally, my doctor suggested that I get counseling to help me work out my feelings and my grief. I guess you can say I did. We now have two adopted children, but I never will be able to put away the memories of the other children who were never to be. I think of them on Christmas. I think of how old they would be and what they would be doing. I don't think anyone could even begin to understand how completely devastating that experience can be.

WARNING SIGNS OF MISCARRIAGE

Miscarriages usually begin with vaginal bleeding, followed by low abdominal cramping that increases with time. Mothers may notice that their early signs of pregnancy, such as tenderness and swelling of the breasts, nausea, and fatigue disappear. If the mother was used to feeling her baby moving, she may notice that the movements have stopped. Listening for the baby's heartbeat and finding none is the final determination that the baby is dead. The expulsion of the fetus can take place any time from a few hours after the mother experiences these signs or symptoms to weeks after the death occurs.

When the fetus dies in the mother's uterus during the first 20 weeks of pregnancy but is not immediately expelled, it is called a *missed abortion.* The mother then faces two choices: to wait for her labor to start spontaneously, or to have her labor induced medically. Most mothers and physicians prefer to have the labor induced; even so, some mothers may wish to wait a few days to become accustomed to the idea of their loss and to say "farewell" to their babies.

MULTIPLE MISCARRIAGE

All parents who experience a miscarriage want to know what the chances are that it will happen again. There are several variables. If it occurs early in pregnancy, the miscarriage was probably caused by random factors, and the risk that it might happen again is small. Even a second miscarriage may have been caused by random factors. However, when a woman has three or more consecutive miscarriages there are probably other factors involved and her opportunity for a successful pregnancy is greatly reduced. She should seek the help of a gynecological specialist to find the source of the problem.

CAUSES OF MISCARRIAGE

Although most parents first blame themselves and then their medical attendants, nature is the main underlying cause in most miscarriages. In reality chromosomal, hormonal, metabolic, and uterine/cervical disorders are the greatest causes for the expulsion of the fetus. Such early miscarriages are usually due to chromosomal abnormalities within the embryo, or abnormalities in the process of implantation. The chromosomal abnormalities may have been caused by a genetic disorder, but most often the cause is in random chance.

Late miscarriages (from the 13th to the 20th week) are usually caused by problems in attachment of the placenta to the uterus, due to abnormalities in the structure of the uterus. Miscarriage may also be caused by a cervix that is weak or incompetent, or one that dilates too early.

Miscarriage can follow a serious disease or infection in the mother. It may also be brought on by malnutrition during pregnancy, smoking, alcohol consumption, and medications. Recent research shows that exposure to environmental and occupational hazards and exposure to radiation also may increase the risk of miscarriage.

Unfortunately, in many miscarriages it is not possible to

determine the specific cause, and the parents are left without a reason.

OVA/SPERM DEFECTS

RANDOM GROSS CHROMOSOMAL ABNORMALITIES

The single most common cause of early miscarriage (before or during implantation) is chromosomal or genetic abnormality. Most of these genetic abnormalities arise from random factors while the ovum and sperm cells (sex cells) are forming in their reproductive cycle. Every human being carries some defective sex cells with gross chromosomal genetic abnormalities. Because of the precarious and delicate process of attaining a healthy human being from the genetic blueprint contained in the single fertilized cell, it is quite a wonder that any fertilized cell makes it through to birth.

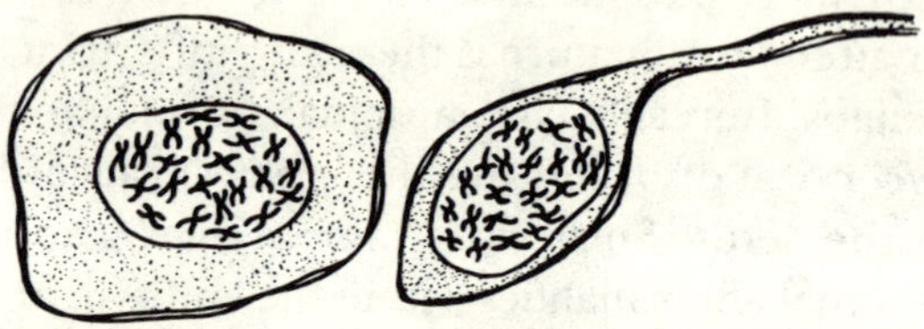

Sex Cells

The immature sex cell itself, whether a sperm or an egg, may carry within it chromosomal abnormalities with genetic misinformation that could not sustain life. In the complex process of dividing and duplicating during mitosis (the division of cells), a normal chromosome may become disfigured, may break off, or another may drift over and attach itself to an already existing pair, scrambling the information and incapacitating it for the support of human life. This type of random chromosomal accident accounts for more than one quarter of early miscarriages.

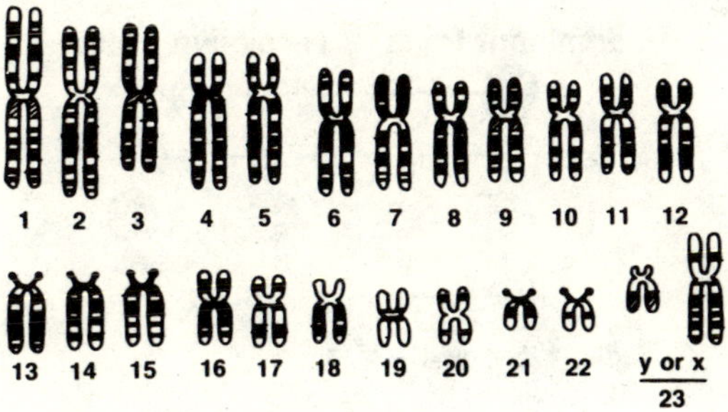

Human Chromosomes

The fertilized egg, in this case, simply does not have the information it needs to produce a healthy human being.

Most of the miscarriages caused by this type of chromosomal abnormality end very early in pregnancy. The earlier in pregnancy the miscarriage takes place, the more likely chromosomal factors have caused it.

Hope for future pregnancies: Because the parent is able to produce normal cells, a random chromosomal abnormality is not likely to be repeated. Future pregnancies will probably not be threatened and the parents, although they may still be anxious, can conceive again.

INHERITED GENETIC DISORDERS

Many human genetic disorders are never visible because they are carried in recessive genes. When chromosomes from the mother and father line up, a recessive gene carried by one parent is covered by the dominant gene of the other parent. So the recessive trait may not be visible, but it is still there to be carried on to future generations. If both the mother and the father carry the recessive gene, there is no dominant gene to cover up the recessive trait, and it may be evident in the offspring.

There are many different types of inherited recessive traits, and they are governed by specific genes. In some instances if

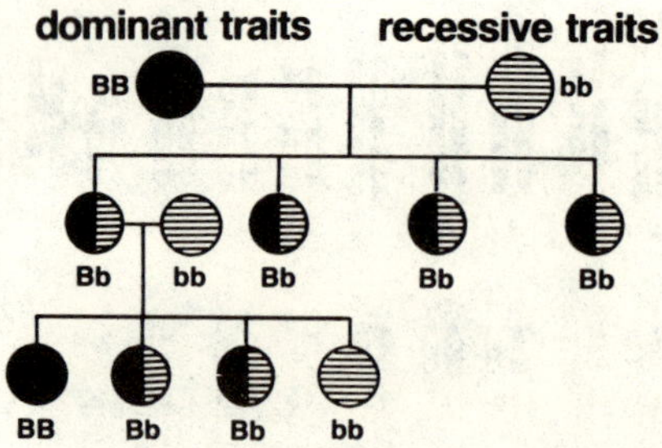

Inheritance

both the mother and father are carriers of a recessive trait, there is a 50 percent likelihood of all their offspring inheriting that trait. In other cases, the chance of the trait being visible in the offspring may be 25 percent or less. Some of these traits, such as hemophilia or color blindness, are not life-threatening to the infant. However, traits such as spina bifida or trisomy 23 are life-threatening, and the fetus will probably be aborted or will die soon after birth.

Hope for future pregnancies: Genetic testing is a diagnostic procedure that can reveal the genetic chromosomal abnormalities in the fetus. With such testing a genetic specialist can help counsel parents if a genetic abnormality does exist and reassure them if it doesn't. Parents can explore what the risks are that such a genetic abnormality might exist in future pregnancies and to what extent. Parents can be helped to make informed choices about the alternatives and options open to them. Community service organizations such as the March of Dimes and Hospice organizations can give valuable information and assistance.

IMPLANTATION DIFFICULTIES

UTERINE ABNORMALITIES

Since implantation usually takes place within six days after conception, many miscarriages occur without anybody even knowing that a fertilized egg was struggling for survival. Miscarriages occur frequently during the complicated process of implantation. If the fertilized egg has chosen a place of implantation on the back wall of the uterus near the top, its chances of survival are great. If, however, the implantation takes place in the lower part of the uterus near the cervix, the placenta can become detached and the fetus may be expelled prematurely.

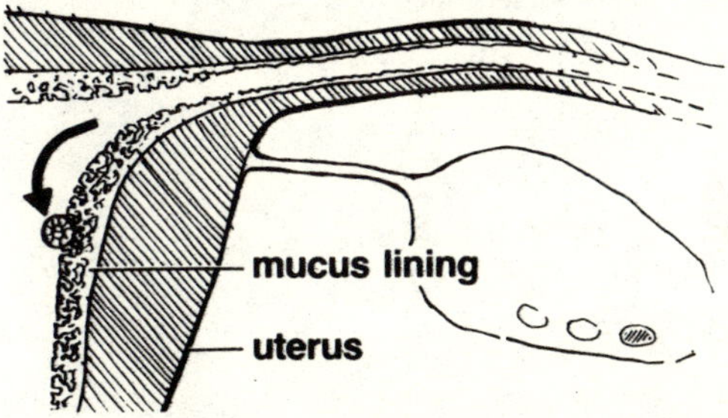

Implantation—Sixth Day

If the uterus is malformed, implantation may be more difficult and the egg may be expelled. If there are fibroid tumors (nonmalignant tumors) the egg may have a difficult or impossible task to implant itself.

Hope for future pregnancies: In the case of random unsuccessful implantation sites, the next pregnancy is not affected. Surgical procedures may be able to correct a malformed uterus and remove fibroid tumors.

INSUFFICIENT PROGESTERONE

If there is inadequate production of progesterone, or if there is an insufficient buildup of the endometrial lining, implantation is impossible. The egg, unable to find a home, is aborted spontaneously.

Hope for future pregnancies: Hormonal therapy may increase chances for successful implantation.

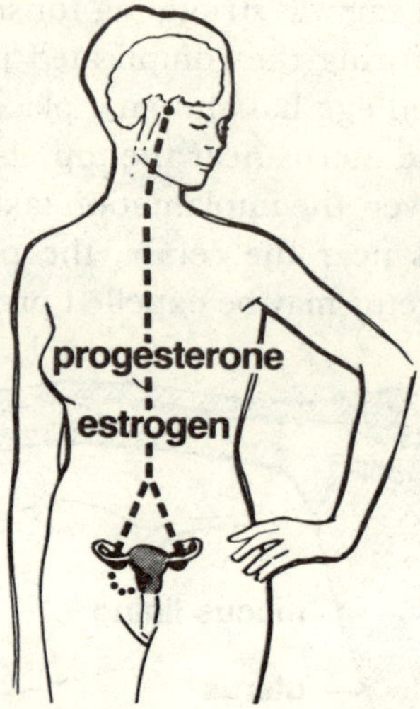

Hormonal Changes

ECTOPIC PREGNANCY

In an especially frustrating experience to a small number of parents, the fertilized egg implants itself outside the uterine cavity, usually in the fallopian tube. Called an ectopic pregnancy, it usually occurs because of previous scarring or infection in the fallopian tubes. Sometime within the first twelve weeks, the developing egg erodes or erupts through the wall of the tube or aborts through its open end. The egg and great quantities of blood flow into the abdominal cavity, causing severe pain and vaginal spotting. If the mother loses a lot of blood she is likely to go into shock. Treatment includes the surgical removal of the tube and blood transfusions.

Hope for future pregnancies: With the removal of the tube, the mother's chances for conceiving future babies may be diminished, but many women still conceive and maintain pregnancies to full term as the remaining ovary takes over.

INABILITY TO MAINTAIN PREGNANCY

UTERINE ABNORMALITIES

Some women are born with abnormalities of the uterus, or there may be scars or adhesions on the uterine wall caused by earlier surgery or infection, which prevent the fertilized egg from implanting. In place of the normally developed uterus, a woman may have two small uteri leading to one common cervix, or two uteri each complete with its own cervix. There may be a wall within the uterus.

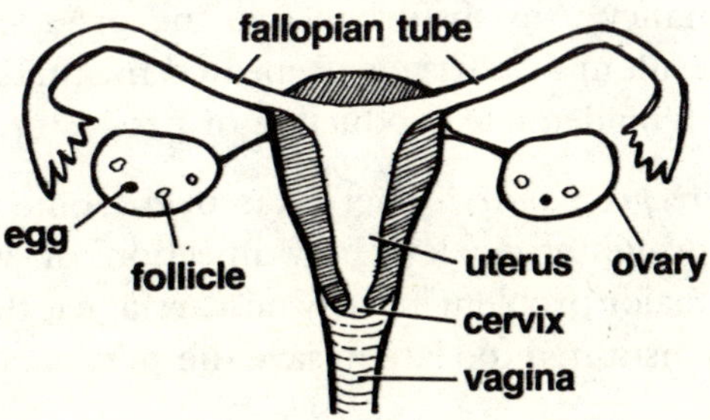

Reproductive System

It is not uncommon to have benign fibroid tumors within the uterus. These are usually not serious and rarely cause other problems, but their position may hamper implantation.

Hope for future pregnancies: These conditions can usually be treated surgically for future pregnancies.

INCOMPETENT CERVIX

Should anything go wrong with the cervix, the fetus or embryo may be expelled unexpectedly at any time. The muscles of the cervix may not be able to hold the baby in if weakened by previous surgical operations (such as induced abortion or D and Cs) or labor. Some cervixes may also be congenitally underdeveloped and the pressure exerted by the increasingly heavy uterus may start dilation.

Hope for future pregnancies: The muscles of the cervix can be reinforced with surgical material wrapped around the cervix like purse strings. These structures are left in place during the pregnancy and are easily removed, to avoid rupturing the uterus, when the mother goes into labor.

INSUFFICIENT SUPPLY OF HORMONES

Progesterone plays a vital role in preserving the life of the embryo during the first two or three months of pregnancy. Estrogen and other hormones are also responsible for maintaining a healthy pregnancy. Any disturbance in the production of hormones may result in miscarriage. Repeated miscarriages may be associated with inadequate production of progesterone.

Hope for future pregnancies: There has been some progress in raising low progesterone levels by injection or vaginal suppositories. A major problem in early miscarriage is that the treatment is often instituted too late to save the pregnancy.

METABOLIC DISTURBANCES

TOXEMIA

If a mother's blood pressure rises, it may be caused by constricted blood vessels and so the blood supply to the baby may be seriously reduced. High blood pressure can be a warning of serious disease such as toxemia. Little is understood about the cause, but the symptoms and results are well known. With toxemia, the mother's blood pressure rises, her kidneys may malfunction, and her hands, feet, and face may swell. Severe and persistent headache, visual disturbance, dizziness or spots before the eyes, marked irritability, and any kind of severe pain in the abdomen are other signs of toxemia. The disease in its extreme stages can be fatal to the baby and can cause convulsions in the mother.

Hope for future pregnancies: With early and good prenatal care, toxemia can be prevented. Women with poor nutrition and those under great stress are the more likely candidates for toxemia. Good nutrition with lots of protein and fluids, and rest and relaxation are preventive measures for toxemia. The expectant mother may be hospitalized if the symptoms become untenable.

DIABETES MELLITUS

Mothers who have diabetes experience a high incidence of miscarriage. Diabetes is the body's inability to process carbohydrates, which are then often present as sugar in the urine. Untreated pregnancies of diabetics usually end in spontaneous abortion. Carried to term, they often result in stillbirths, neonatal deaths, or the delivering of abnormal infants. Pregnancy, acting as a stress factor, may precipitate or predispose a woman to diabetes.

Hope for future pregnancies: For the first time in history, depending on the class and severity of the disease, women with diabetes have the chance to carry their babies to healthy births through medical intervention and monitoring by obstetricians and internists.

THYROID DISORDERS

Although there is some disagreement as to the effects of hyperthyroidism on pregnancy, most doctors feel that uncontrolled hyperthyroidism leads to miscarriage and fetal or neonatal death.

Hope for future pregnancies: When the disease is medically controlled the outcome can be quite successful.

OTHER FACTORS

Miscarriages are more prevalent in women who have been exposed during pregnancy to German measles (rubella), herpes simplex virus number 2, measles, mumps, polio, chicken pox, and hepatitis. There is also a higher risk of miscarriage for women who have some heart conditions, have kidney disease, or who suffer from extremely high blood pressure.

3

Stillbirth

Parents who experience a stillbirth are not only faced with the death of their babies, but have had the pain, effort, and expense of labor and delivery. The irony of working through each contraction of labor, of enduring transition, of pushing out their dead child, and producing a lifeless infant symbolizes the special tragedy of stillbirth.

DEFINITION OF STILLBIRTH

When a fetus dies between the 20th week of pregnancy and birth, it is called a stillbirth. The baby dies while still in the mother's uterus, but the parents may not be aware of this until labor is under way or the birth takes place. For every live 1,000 births there are 12.6 stillbirths.

CHRISTY AND JAMES

STILLBIRTH AT 38 WEEKS

When I became pregnant it was like all of our dreams were going to come true at once. My pregnancy was very normal. I was huge but otherwise felt terrific. It was really a wonderful time for me. I felt like I looked really terrific. I enjoyed it thoroughly, which makes me feel good now.

About my thirty-eighth week of pregnancy, I developed toxemia. The doctor told me he was going to put me in the hospital and that he would either induce me if my symptoms didn't reverse themselves, or if they did, he would let me carry it to term. As soon as I went into the hospital my symptoms began to reverse themselves, I started to lose weight, I didn't have protein in my urine any more, my blood pressure went down, and everything was looking really good. He was going to send me home the following day, and he asked the nurses to do some tests.

About noon the first two nurses came in and turned the machine on and hooked everything up, and nothing happened. They just said, "Oh, the machine's on the fritz." They got another one and tried it, and—nothing. The nurse started looking around for a heartbeat, and I remember looking at one of them and saying, "Should I be upset?" I really thought they were going to find a heartbeat because sometimes in the doctor's office he would have to search a little bit before he could find it. But by this time there were about half a dozen nurses in the room, and then the head nurse came in, and I remember looking up into her face and she had tears in her eyes. I knew then. One of the nurses flew out of the room and flew back in with the doctor. He came with his little shower cap and his booties. He was very straightforward and told me right away, "I don't think the baby is alive."

They scheduled me for an ultrasound, and that confirmed his suspicions. He came back about an hour and a half later and induced me with a suppository. About dinnertime, I remember having very strong contractions. From the onset, they were about a minute or a minute and a half apart. It was all just kind of a blur. The doctor came back at about seven and broke my water. About an hour later I had the urge to push. I had my husband get the nurse. I delivered about a half hour later. The doctor was just walking in and the baby was crowning, and then she was born. I had terrible fears that there must be something hideously wrong. "Why did she die? Everything was okay, wasn't it?" I asked my husband, "Was it a boy?" He said, "No, honey, it was a beautiful little girl." The doctor administered a sedative, and I slept for a while. James saw the baby and held her and cried over her.

KATHERINE AND LARRY

STILLBIRTH AT 40 WEEKS

I was very excited when I got pregnant. It was something I wanted and everything was going along just wonderfully. One week prior to my due date, everything looked just great when I went for my regular weekly doctor's visit. My chart looked just like a model chart should: perfect blood pressure, perfect urine sample tests, perfect blood tests, everything was just perfect. I remember every detail of that day. I remember lying down and joking with the nurse about the baby while the doctor was listening for the baby's heartbeat. He started using his hand and I started to get a little worried. He left the room and came in with the Doppler monitor.

The longer and longer he searched, the less he said. It started to dawn on me that the baby was dead. I remember the doctor saying, "I'm really concerned." Finally he said, "I just don't know what to say to you. There was nothing to indicate that there would be anything wrong, but I just can't find a heartbeat. We're going to send you down to ultrasound to make sure."

I remember looking at the baby's picture and the doctor saying, "There's the head, there's the feet," and he said "Now this is the heart." It seemed like forever before he said, "I'm sorry," and walked out of the room. I just remember screaming. I wanted my husband, I wanted to call my husband. I thought, "I'm going to go crazy, I've got to have some help. Oh, my God, now I've got to go through labor. I shouldn't have to go through labor and delivery." After all those months of being positive, I was just totally negative. I said, "I don't want to feel anything or see anything, just knock me out."

When we got to the hospital my husband was there. I didn't want him to touch me. I couldn't even stand to touch myself because it was a reminder that the baby was dead. It was so hideous to think that he was dead and still inside of me. I just wanted to get him out. They gave me some drugs and inserted a suppository, which was supposed to make me go into labor. The doctor told me what was going to happen and what to expect. I immediately went into labor. I remember thinking, I spent all that time and money and effort to go through Lamaze, I might as well make myself as comfortable as possible.

When the baby was finally born eight hours later, I remember the doctor saying, "I don't know what to say, but I'm sorry." He told me that he was proud of how I went through labor, and I thought, "Well, at least I did something right." I'm glad I wasn't drugged because it was my first baby and I experienced labor and delivery. Now I know that there is nothing to be afraid of. If I can go through labor and delivery knowing that my baby is dead, I can handle anything. After I went home, I felt so bizarre, like I was the only one that this had ever happened to. How was I ever going to explain this to anyone?

WARNING SIGNS OF STILLBIRTH

Some mothers may experience symptoms that signal all is not normal. There may be some bleeding from the vagina or severe cramping and stabbing sensations in the pelvis and lower back or abdomen. Mothers who experience stillbirth may gradually become aware that there has been no movement for more than a day. The doctor will listen for the heartbeat through traditional methods. He may use ultrasound to see the baby and determine if the heart is beating.

SPONTANEOUS AND INDUCED LABOR

When a baby dies in the mother's uterus, the mother usually goes into labor and delivers spontaneously within two weeks of the death. If the labor does not start spontaneously labor should be medically induced before the fourth week after death, because a mother carrying a dead fetus has an increased risk of developing severe blood problems.

Giving the mother and father choices in the decision of when to induce labor may give them some feeling of control in a situation that has left them completely out of control. Some parents may wish to have labor started as soon as possible. Others may wish to carry the baby to a spontaneous labor so that they can have as natural a birth as possible.

CAUSES OF STILLBIRTH

UMBILICAL CORD ACCIDENTS

The umbilical cord, which supplies oxygen and nourishment to the fetus, is the baby's life support system. As the baby moves around, turning and twisting, the cord may develop a kink, or even a knot. As the baby moves down during labor the cord may get squeezed, or it may twist around the baby's neck, resulting in decreasing nourishment and oxygen and finally death. Although cord accidents can happen before labor, most accidents occur during labor and delivery as the baby moves down through the mother's pelvis.

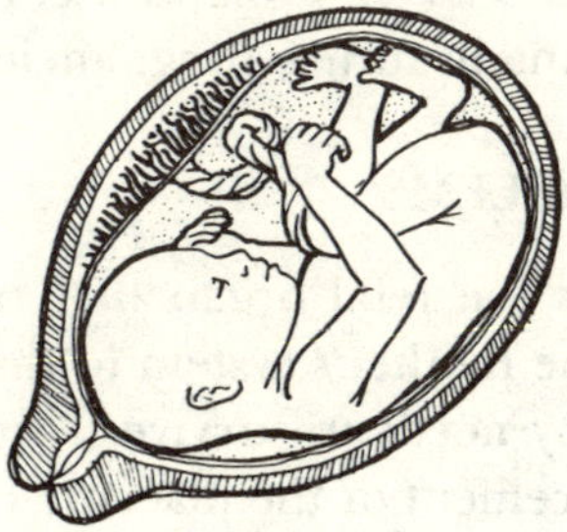

Fetal Development—Seventh Month

Hope for future pregnancies: Umbilical cord accidents have no effect on future pregnancies. Although the parents will never again take birth for granted, they can conceive, bear, and give birth with little risk this accident will happen again.

PROLAPSED CORD

Uterine contraction may force the membranes of the placenta through an incompletely dilated cervix. If these membranes rupture early, the cord may extend past the presenting part of the baby. Once the cord is out of the uterus, and especially when out of the vagina, the baby's blood and oxygen supply is obstructed. As the healthy baby moves down through the mother's pelvis, its body presses against the cord and cuts off the life-giving oxygen supply.

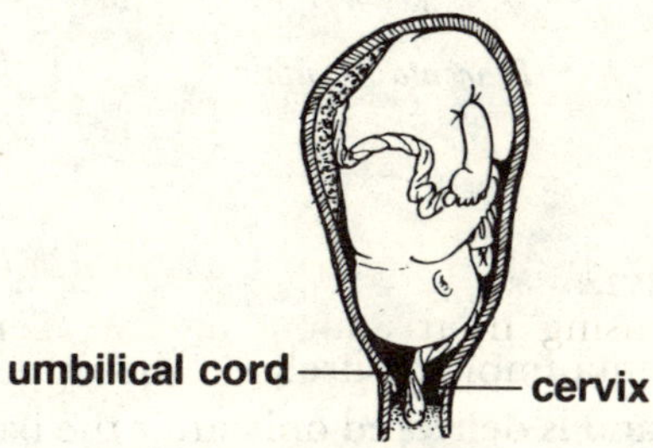

Prolapsed Cord

Hope for future pregnancies: A prolapsed cord accident has little possibility of recurring in future pregnancies.

PLACENTAL PROBLEMS

The placenta is the fetal organ that transforms nutrients and oxygen from the mother's system to the forms of nutrients and oxygen the baby needs to survive. Any problems with the development or placement of the placenta can be disastrous for the baby.

PLACENTA ABRUPTIO

If, during pregnancy, the placenta begins to separate from its implantation site at the wall of the uterus, the supply of nutrients and oxygen to the baby may be diminished. If the placenta separates completely, the baby will not be able to survive. Placenta abruptio brings excruciating uterine pain to the mother with extensive bleeding. The occurrence of separation is most common in the third trimester.

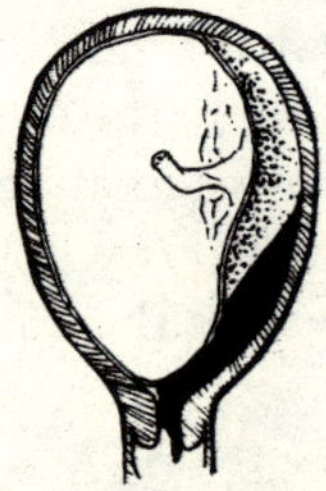

Placenta Abruptio

PLACENTA PREVIA

Normally the placenta implants itself on the upper right-hand side of the uterus, and is delivered only after the baby is born. If the placenta implants itself in the lower portion of the uterus, there may be some bleeding but the baby can survive. If, however, it implants itself over the mouth of the cervix, the placenta will be delivered before the baby, cutting off the oxygen supply and resulting in fetal death.

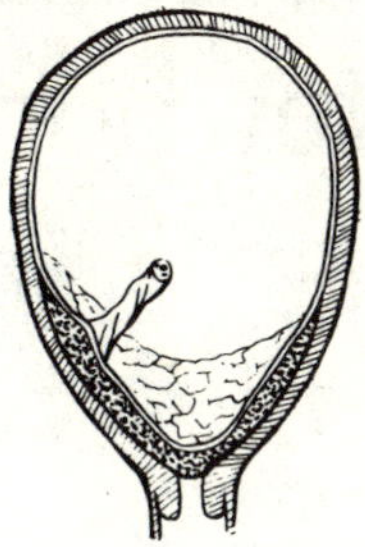

Placenta Previa

Hope for future pregnancies: Because the placenta is an organ formed from the embryonic material, its implantation site is dependent not on the mother's systems but the baby's. The chances of developing successive placenta previa or placenta abruptio conditions are minimal.

ANOXIA

Anoxia, or the cutting off of the fetal oxygen supply, is the major cause of stillbirth incidences. Anoxia is brought on by umbilical cord accidents and placental problems.

OTHER CAUSES

1. Fetal genetic factors and genetic abnormalities;
2. Maternal problems such as toxemia, Rh antigen antibody formation, anemias, infections.

Stillbirth is especially frustrating because there is no known cause for up to one half of all stillbirths.

4

Death of a Newborn

Parents whose babies die soon after birth are faced with the special torment of waiting. Not only do they experience the stresses of labor, but also the paralyzing terror at birth when the medical staff signals that something has gone wrong. There is an unconscious ambivalence about whether to bond to their babies or to separate themselves from the infants. If the baby is transferred to a distant medical center, the situation becomes even more complicated. The uncertainty of waiting, hoping, wishing, and bargaining before the babies die, and then finally going home without the child, is a special tragedy.

JANET AND PAUL

NEWBORN DEATH

I remember going to the first OB visit. I had caught the flu very early in my pregnancy, high temperatures, and the whole bit, and everybody just dismissed it. Probably it didn't have anything to do with it, but there is a certain theory I read in a genetics book that maybe there is some correlation. I remember the first question I asked my doctor during the initial consultation was, "What are the chances of having an abnormal child, a child with Down's syndrome, or something like that?" He said, "You have one normal child. This is the second one, so there is little chance of a problem."

I started labor at 2:00 A.M. and the baby was born by 8:30 A.M. I opened my eyes and I could see this little tiny foot, little tiny hands waving around. Then the doctor said, "There is something wrong with this baby." He rushed over to the little isolette and immediately they started to try to get the baby to breathe. He said, "Oh, my God, call the pediatrician! There is an emergency team here from the children's hospital, get them!" So they came rushing in, four people, and our doctor and the nurse, and they were getting all this stuff into the baby and trying to get her to breathe and then our pediatrician came. We were lying there for about half an hour watching this whole thing and Paul was wrenching my hand off and saying, "Come on, come on, little baby, be okay." One of the nurses kept coming over and touching my hand, trying to give us some information about what was happening.

Finally, I looked at the clock and I asked, "Do you know how long it's been?" "It's been almost a half an hour," Paul said.

"Even if she lives, what's the use?" So we said, "Would you stop, would you please stop?" The children's hospital team looked at us like, "Those people are insane, who let them out of the wacko ward?" We said again, "Stop," and our doctor, our OB, picked it up from there and he said, "Yes, I think there is some problem with this baby that we can't save anyway, so everybody stop." Then there was complete silence. Pretty soon the nurse said, "Didn't anybody even notice what time the baby was born?"

I remember thinking how calm I was because I knew from the beginning that this pregnancy and this baby weren't right, and nobody would listen to me.

RHONDA AND HARRY

NEWBORN DEATH

We went into labor confident and excited. When my water broke, the nurse seemed kind of confused and went to get the doctor. She mentioned that the color was kind of different, but we were so busy with our breathing that I didn't pay much attention. They wheeled in the fetal monitor and I thought that all the special attention we were getting was normal. But now, I remember the concern in their voices.

When we went into delivery, I remembered the movies we had seen and I reminded the doctor that I wanted to hold my baby and nurse him on the delivery table. He said only, "We'll see." I pushed and pushed and finally heard a faint cry. I was surprised when no one said anything. I remember looking up at Harry and he had a strange look on his face. The doctor didn't say anything and the nurse seemed to be waiting. Everybody was concentrating on the baby and as they took him over to the isolette, I noticed something on his back. I asked the doctor what it was. He told me, "Your baby had a little problem. We want to look into it before we talk about it more," and he walked out leaving me and my husband there with a chill in our hearts.

A nurse came and held my hand and told me not to worry. Not to worry? I felt like I was in a nightmare and everything was going slow-motion around me. I think Harry must have felt the same way because I can't remember him saying anything, just holding my hand so hard it hurt. Somehow I got back to my room and we waited. We didn't know it then, but that was just the beginning of waiting: waiting for doctors, for opinions, for nurses, for reports. The pediatrician came in, not our own doctor but a complete stranger, and told us our baby had spina bifida. We were silent, shocked, we didn't know what to say. None of our birth books had talked about spina bifida. I remember drifting in and out while he was explaining that it was a birth defect and that we would talk about it later.

I wanted to see my baby. I didn't care what he looked like, I didn't care if he was a monster, I wanted to see and hold my baby. I remember being surprised by the intensity of my emotions. I think I would have fought tigers and all if they had stood in my way. The nurse took me into the nursery and let me look at him. He wasn't a monster; he was a little angel and he was mine.

Later on, the nurses asked me if I wanted to breast-feed my baby and they showed me how to pump my milk and bring it in. He died the next day but I will always be glad that I was able to give my milk to him. It made me feel that I had really mothered him and done the best I could; I will never have any regrets, and I'll always be thankful to the nurses who helped and encouraged me.

When Michael died, I was devastated. I knew intellectually that he would not live, but I hoped emotionally that he would. I really feel though, that the little time I had with him, holding him, touching him, giving him my milk—all these made my grieving a little easier. I think my husband and I both want to go on now and have another baby. Not to replace Michael, but to add to our family.

SANDY AND CHARLES

EARLY INFANT DEATH

It had been a difficult pregnancy, not at all like my first one. I had had spotting and just didn't feel well through the whole pregnancy. One morning in the beginning of the sixth month, my water broke. I was shocked—I knew it was too early, and I was worried that my baby would never survive this early in his development. I called my neighbor and she took me to the hospital. When I arrived, I was in full labor and knew that there was no way we could turn back. My neighbor had called my husband and he was there at the emergency room. There was no time for anything, it was all just frantic. Before I knew it I was pushing down. When the baby was born, there was no joy, no telling me I had a beautiful baby boy, just silence. My husband held my hand and I knew something was terribly wrong. I was afraid to ask him and I think he was afraid to say anything to me.

They rushed the baby out into an ambulance and to another hospital where the nurse said that there would be special equipment and he would get the best care. It was all like a dream. I didn't get to see him until three days later. He had tubes and cords in every opening in his body. I still felt paralyzed and moved through life as if it were all a dream and I would wake up later.

I felt totally helpless. I would watch my baby, watch his chest rise and fall, watch each breath as a courageous effort and there was nothing I could do. I felt guilty because of the new baby. I felt guilty because I didn't have the energy to give my daughter at home any comfort or mothering even though I knew she needed me. I couldn't give my husband the emotional comfort he needed. The baby died after sixteen days of struggle and pain. It helped me so much that the hospital staff had let me hold him and feed him. But my arms still ached with the loneliness.

Charles could hardly go to the hospital those days. He didn't want to talk about it. He only buried himself in his work. Then he wanted to get over it right away. Wanted to have another baby right away. I kept trying to get over it, kept trying to do and say the right things, but when my baby died, a part of me died too. There is still a place in my heart that is dead, and I think it will always be there.

The autopsy showed that our baby had genetic abnormalities. When we went in to talk about future babies, we found that we had a 25 percent chance of repeating this experience. I just don't feel up to it now. My first child gives me a lot of joy and courage. I know we'll try again. But it's going to take some time to get my strength again.

CAUSES OF NEWBORN DEATH

The major factors contributing to a newborn death are:

1. Premature birth,
2. Postmature birth,
3. Rh sensitization factors,
4. Fetal distress,
5. Genetic chromosomal abnormalities,
6. Intrauterine infection,
7. Inability of a marginally healthy baby to withstand the stress of labor and delivery,
8. Overlapping factors such as prematurity, maternal hormonal deficiency, maternal disease, congenital deformities (that is, heart disease or respiratory failure).

PREMATURE BIRTH

One of the leading causes of newborn death is the birth of a baby before his or her systems are mature enough to sustain life outside of his or her mother's body. Today, medical care can allow many premature babies to live a normal, healthy life. However, many other babies with immature respiratory and other vital systems cannot survive. Although 1 percent of all births are twins, 10 percent of all premature deaths occur in twin and

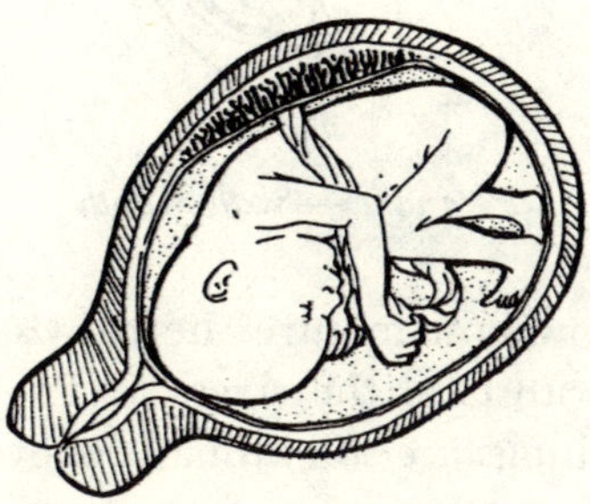

Fetal Development—Fifth Month

multiple births. When one twin survives and the other does not the parents are caught in an especially painful role of grieving for the one and trying to attach to and nurture the other. Because premature births are always early and unexpected they create special stresses for the parents.

Hope for future pregnancies: Because premature babies are often small for their gestational age, they are the most compromised and have the lowest survival rate of all babies. When a woman begins a premature labor, medical treatment is administered to stop or delay labor in order to prolong the gestation of the pregnancy. Although no one really knows what starts labor, research is being done on drugs that help arrest premature labor by inhibiting the contractions of the uterus.

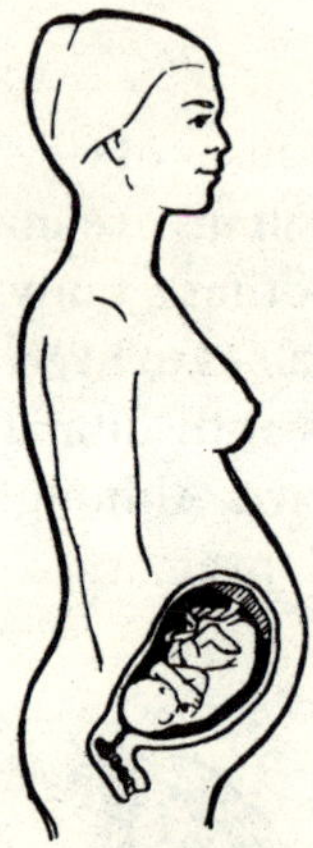

Pregnancy—Sixth Month

Tests now show how mature the baby's lungs are, and if they are able to withstand the stresses of labor and delivery. Particularly if the lungs are still immature, every effort is made to sustain the pregnancy.

Hyaline membrane disease is one of the leading killers of premature infants. Because of a deficiency of a pulmonary surface agent (a natural detergentlike substance in the respiratory passages of the lungs), the passages become clogged and the baby cannot breathe. Research is developing corticosteroid drugs that can promote the maturation of the baby's lungs.

POSTMATURITY

There is some indication that there is a relationship between postmaturity and fetal distress and mortality. Certain congenital anomalies cause the pregnancy to progress beyond the 42-week gestation. As the placenta ages, its capacity to supply oxygen and nutrients to the baby is reduced. This weakens the baby's ability to cope with the stress of labor and delivery. Although the baby may appear normal, dry peeling skin indicates the lack of a lubricating cream that is normally present during pregnancy.

Hope for future pregnancies: Doctors are now using fetal assessment tools for the baby's lung maturity, and the placental output to determine the time of conception and the optimum delivery date. If the woman proceeds past that date, the baby can be delivered safely by inducing labor or by cesarean childbirth.

Rh SENSITIZATION FACTORS

In 13 percent of all marriages, the mother's blood lacks a certain factor (Rh) that the father's blood includes. If the baby

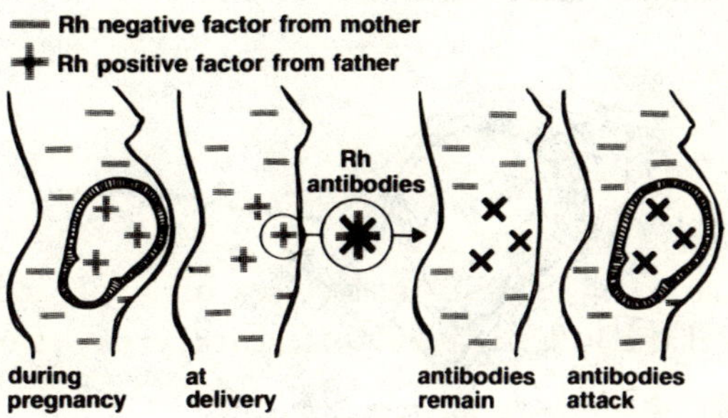

Rh Factor

inherits the father's factor (Rh-positive) and the mother has Rh-negative blood during pregnancy, the mother's body may react to her baby's blood type and develop antibodies against that type. Her first Rh-positive baby will not be affected, although the antibodies she had developed will affect subsequent Rh-positive pregnancies, which may result in msicarriage, stillbirth, or necessitate blood transfusions at birth. The mother will, of course, have no problem if her baby has her own Rh-negative factor.

Hope for future pregnancies: Today mothers can receive gamma globulin that will counteract her body's natural inclination to develop antibodies during her pregnancy. This allows her to carry her future pregnancies to term.

FETAL DISTRESS

During birth, the baby's passage through the birth canal is a hazardous journey. Throughout the labor, the baby's heart tones indicate how he or she is responding to the rigors of contractions and may signal a decrease in oxygen supply from the placenta. Sometimes the contractions and length of labor can be so stressful that a baby, especially one that is in marginal health, cannot survive.

Hope for future pregnancies: If the reasons for fetal distress are accidental, then recurrence is rare. If the causes for fetal distress

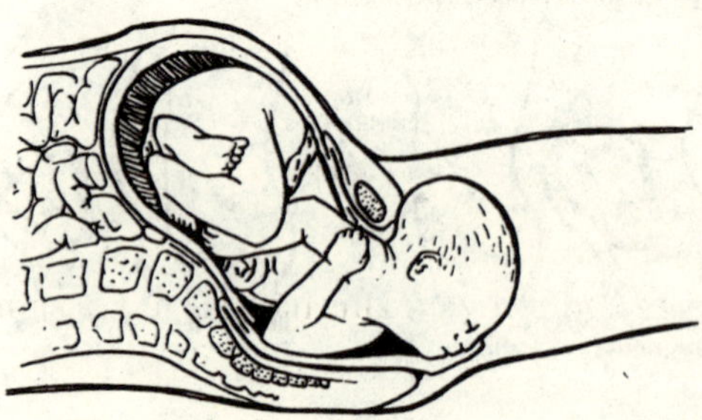

Expulsion (extension)

are genetic abnormalities, then the risk for recurring fetal distress in subsequent pregnancies is greater. With modern medical equipment, the baby's ability to withstand stress can be constantly monitored. A cesarean delivery for a compromised baby may avert disaster.

GENETIC CHROMOSOMAL ABNORMALITIES

If a child with gross genetic abnormalities survives for a time after birth, the parents suffer a double pain. They may be embarrassed and self-conscious about producing a deformed baby. They have no idea how to react or what to do. Many terrible thoughts about the appearance of the baby occur to the parents before they see the child: "Will he be a monster?" They may suffer guilt and feelings of failure. At the same time they experience ambivalent feelings of love and affection for their baby.

Hope for future pregnancies: If the baby carries chromosomal abnormalities that affect the development of its vital systems, genetic studies can be done to determine if either one of the parents or the fetus carries the abnormal chromosomal defect. If the abnormality is through random chance, the parents can conceive, carry, and give birth to a future healthy baby with relatively more confidence that if the abnormality is genetic. If genetic, it is advisable to receive genetic counseling before making a decision to conceive another child. Genetic counseling can give parents some idea of what the odds are for the abnormality to be repeated. Amniocentesis is another diagnostic tool which can be used to detect chromosomal abnormalities in the fetus.

DIAGNOSTIC TESTING TECHNIQUES DURING PREGNANCY

Every couple's hope is for a normal, healthy baby. Just because a couple experienced a miscarriage, stillbirth, or newborn death, it does not mean that they are doomed to repeat the experience.

New techniques are now used to determine how well the unborn baby is doing in the uterine environment. Tests have been designed to help determine the due date, the baby's maturity, the baby's well-being, the efficiency of the placenta, the baby's ability to withstand the stresses of labor and delivery. Techniques have also been developed to help couples who face genetic risks. It is important that parents understand both the benefits and risks of diagnostic testing.

AMNIOCENTESIS

The amniotic fluid surrounding the baby contains cells that give important information concerning the unborn baby. A sample of this fluid is extracted in the technique called *amniocentesis,* which can be performed either in a hospital or in an out-patient setting.

The mother's abdomen is scrubbed and a sterile needle inserted through the abdomen and uterus into the amniotic sac from which the fluid is withdrawn. In early pregnancy, cultures can be made from the cells and tests run that can diagnose genetic disorders such as Down's syndrome, sex-linked diseases, or the severity of Rh disease. By this test the baby's sex can also be determined.

Later in pregnancy, amniocentesis can be performed to determine the maturity of the baby's lungs, should either the baby's or the mother's condition indicate that the baby should be born as soon as possible. If the baby is born before his or her lungs are mature, he or she has a greater chance of developing hyaline membrane disease and respiratory distress—the leading cause of neonatal death.

OXYTOCIN CHALLENGE TEST

If the mother develops diabetes or other complications, the Oxytocin Challenge Test (O.C.T.) is used to determine how the baby and the placenta react to the contractions of labor and whether labor must be initiated for the mother's or baby's sake. Before labor begins, the woman is given a synthetic hormone (oxytocin) to stimulate contractions of the uterus. At the same time, the mother and baby are connected to a fetal monitor that makes a continuous recording of the baby's heart rate and the mother's uterine contractions. If the baby's heart rate drops significantly after contractions, it is assumed that the baby is in danger. If the heart rate does not show a drop after each contraction, the fetus can remain in the uterus for further development.

ALPHA-FETOPROTEIN (AFP) MEASUREMENTS

Alpha-fetoprotein, a substance produced by the baby, can be measured in the amniotic fluid and from samples of the mother's blood during pregnancy. High levels of this protein indicate a likelihood of brain and spinal-cord abnormalities.

ESTRIOL

Estriol is an estrogen product formed jointly by the placenta and the fetus. The level of estriol in the mother's blood or urine tells how well the placenta is functioning in providing oxygen and nutrients to her baby. Estriol levels rise as the pregnancy progresses, reflecting the normal growth of the baby. Since estriol levels vary, the mother's urine is tested several times in a twenty-four-hour period.

ULTRASOUND

Ultrasound helps establish the baby's age as well as the possibility of a multiple birth. It also locates the placenta (for amniocentesis) and can identify any gross abnormalities. In ultrasound high-frequency sound waves are sent through the mother's abdomen and placenta to the baby. Echoes of the sound waves bounce back and are translated onto an oscilloscope showing either a still or moving picture of the fetus. When these pictures are taken over a period of time, they can help determine intrauterine growth and estimate the due date.

ELECTRONIC FETAL MONITOR

The fetal monitor is an important tool in high-risk pregnancies, labors, and deliveries. The presence of fetal distress, when the baby suffers from insufficient circulation of blood from the placenta or compression of the umbilical cord, is detected by use of the fetal monitor. The baby's heart rate reveals whether he or she is receiving sufficient oxygen from the placenta. If the oxygen drops, the baby's heart rate drops.

The fetal monitor also measures the baby's capacity to withstand the uterine contractions of labor. In the past, the nurse or medical caregiver could only monitor the progress of the labor by timing and evaluating the mother's contractions, and by listening to the baby's heart through a stethoscope. The electronic fetal monitor records on a paper graph the baby's heartbeat as it relates to the frequency, length, and strength of the uterine contractions. The monitor also records at the same time the variations of acceleration (speeding up) and deceleration (slowing down) that exist in relationship to the uterine contractions. An irregular heartbeat (deceleration) with contractions may indicate that the baby is in trouble and measures should be taken to increase the oxygen supply or speed up the birth (that is, cesarean).

II

Grief

5

The Loss

Since doctors and nurses are the first people present when the death of a baby occurs, the reactions and the quality of care they provide make an enormous difference in how the parents will cope with their tragedy. Probably the most important thing the staff can do is to let the parents know that the feelings they are experiencing are not only normal but appropriate. They should provide a nonthreatening and nonjudgmental atmosphere where the parents can express their thoughts and questions openly and be supported by an understanding and compassionate staff. With parents who do not know how to show their grief, or who don't have a support system of family or friends, it may take more time and effort to let them know that talking, crying, and yelling are all acceptable and important expressions of grief.

TELLING THE PARENTS OF THE DEATH

The first and major task of the staff is to tell the parents the baby has died or will die. How this news is initially presented has tremendous consequences for the final resolution of grief. If the news is broken in brief medical terminology parents are left with frustration and ignorance and long-term negative feelings. Those parents who are informed in a sensitive and nontechnical manner by their physician of the death or impending death of the baby are in a better position to work through their grief and have some positive memories of the experience.

The mother and father need to be together when the doctor informs them of the condition of their child. They need to hear reassuring statements that they are not failures, and that this does not necessarily mean the end of their parenthood. They need to hear about the positive aspects of the pregnancy and birth; to be told what a good job they did during labor and delivery. They need to see the perfections in their baby.

A sensitive staff does not just explain what happened once, but returns frequently, checking on the couple and repeating what the couple needs to hear again. As grief progresses, parents are able to hear and integrate more facts. They are able to articulate questions. The best explanation is factual, compassionate, and free of technical jargon. If the baby was born alive but there is good reason to believe he or she will die, the doctor should explain in plain language what the problem is. It is important that the parents understand that no matter what is going to happen, everything will be done to support both the baby and themselves.

"I remember very clearly—my doctor all through this said, 'I don't know what to say to you. I'm very sorry, but I don't know what to say.' And I think it was really good that he didn't use a lot of clichés. He just kept saying 'I don't know what to say, but I'm sorry.' And to me, that statement was the one that most people who were really honest about the whole thing said. 'I don't know what to say, but I'm sorry that it happened to you.'"

"When the baby was dying one nurse was constantly coming over and telling us what was happening. She broke down and cried with us at the end."

"Every mother I have talked to vividly remembers details of the events surrounding the loss. It is important for the staff to know that everything they say and do we remember with great clarity."

"I think one of the first things that I needed reassuring on was that I was going to be OK physically. I had a feeling of doom, like, the baby is dead, now I'm going to die, too. And it was helpful when the doctor told me 'Well, you're going to be all right, and you're going to recover.' "

"My doctor said to me, 'This is one of the most difficult things you are ever going to have to do or that anybody can go through, and you've survived it, and I want you to know that I'm proud of you, the way that you've handled yourself, and your attitude.' That made me feel really good."

CHOICES IN THE HOSPITAL

When a baby dies, parents feel completely out of control and vulnerable to the vagaries of fate. Responsibility for the many decisions that have to be made immediately following the death has a great impact on the parents. It is very important to be given a choice of whether to see or hold the baby, whether to have photographs taken, whether to give the baby a name.

Having the pros and cons of an autopsy explained and being included in the disposition of the baby's body and funeral arrangements can give parents a sense of regaining control. This is important in the initial attempts to deal with loss.

"The chance to make a decision should be given to you several times. I know I was so dopey that a decision that I made the first day was very different from the one I would make the second. So the staff shouldn't take your first decision, but give you a second chance."

"Being given options makes it a lot easier to make the right choices. The wrong decisions that are made at this time can later lead to guilt. Like I didn't see my baby, and I feel guilty about it now. Or, looking back, I should have given my baby a name. That can go on for years and years. It seems the guilt is always there. It's not something to be taken lightly."

SEEING AND HOLDING THE BABY

One of the earliest decisions that faces parents is whether or not to see the baby. It is important that the staff let the parents know that they have the option to see and hold their baby.

Research shows that viewing, touching, and holding the baby helps parents to work through their grief. Mothers and fathers who have seen their dead infants seem to have an easier time accepting and coping with grief. Seeing the baby brings the reality of death to them. It helps to reaffirm that they gave birth and are the parents of a baby. Seeing the baby also gives a concrete image to share with others. And, if there are deformities, seeing the baby is generally far less painful for the parents than not seeing him or her and imagining the deformities.

It is equally important to recognize that if the decision to see the child is forced on the parents they will regret it with the same intensity as parents who are not given this option. Accept the couple's final decision—different people have the right to different opinions and needs. Their control over their decision is as important as the decision they make.

The parents should be given as much time as they want to be with their baby, to say their good-byes. They should be able to decide whether they want the nurse or doctor to stay with them or whether they want to be alone.

PREPARATION

The staff should prepare the couple for what they will see. They should be gently told that the baby's body may feel cold or unresponsive. Parents are often surprised that their dead baby looks like one who is sleeping. Even if the baby is deformed, parents can usually see something special or perfect in him or her. If there are deformities, the nurse can bring the baby to the mother wrapped in a blanket with the deformities covered. She can point out the perfect fingers or the perfect ears. If the baby has been dead in the uterus for some time, the parents should be prepared for the color of the baby. And, if there are lacerations or deformations of the skin, the nurse should explain them and their causes.

> "I was really afraid to see my baby because they told me that due to abnormalities caused by chromosomal syndrome the baby was deformed. I thought of a monster—I had given birth to a monster. But, I decided that it was my baby and that I wanted to see her. When they brought her to me all wrapped in a little blanket, I saw a sleeping doll. She had the most perfect fingers. I touched them and marveled at their perfection. I will always remember my baby and holding her sweet fingers in mine will stay with me forever."

"Our obstetrician and pediatrician both advised us not to see the baby. We went along with them. Now we regret that decision. We know that they were acting with best intentions, but even though our baby was deformed nothing could be as bad as our fantasies. I wish now that they would have given us another chance."

NAMING THE BABY

Another choice that confronts parents is whether to name their baby. Those who name their child find they have a concrete person about whom to talk. The name reaffirms that they have had a child; it helps them accept the reality of the death. Naming the child can also help the live children and those born in subsequent pregnancies. It gives each child an identity within the family.

PREPARATION

The parents can choose to use the name they had chosen prior to birth, or, if it was a treasured family name, they can save the original name for another child, and select a special name for the deceased child. Since the parents may be in shock, it is important to point out that they are free to choose another name if they are not comfortable with the original chosen name. Parents should also know that if they choose not to name now, this decision may be altered later.

"When they told me my baby died, I got up and thought for a long time. I realized that if he died it meant he had also lived and he deserved a name. I'm glad we chose to do that because it's important for us to be able to refer to him as Stephen."

"The very first thing we decided when we found out we were pregnant was the name. We were going to name it after our fathers. If it was a boy it was going to be Alexander Dean and if it was a girl it was going to be Alexis Deanne. When we told our fathers, they just thought it was the most wonderful thing in the world. But when the baby died, we couldn't give him that special name we had put away. And so we found another name, Christian, and that was his name. We gave it to him a year later and it was just right."

HAVING THE BABY'S PHOTOGRAPH TAKEN

Another option is whether or not to have the baby's picture taken. Those who have photographs of their babies have a permanent remembrance that reaffirms not only to the parents but to others that there really was a baby and that they really are parents.

"I would like to have a photograph. Maybe not for myself. But there are a few people that I would like to show and say, 'See I really did have a baby.' I could say, 'This is my baby. Wasn't he cute? Wasn't he perfect?' I would like to be able to take it out and reassure myself and say to others, 'Look, you are dismissing this, but here is my baby.'"

COMPLETING OFFICIAL DOCUMENTS

Parents, prepared only for the birth certificate, are shocked and unprepared for the documents of death. It is important that the staff help them through this painful process.

"The greatest shock I had was going to the funeral home and signing the death certificate. When I had to sign my name as the father, the tragedy finally dawned on me. It was the first time I cried."

AUTOPSY

Often the most difficult choice is whether or not to have an autopsy performed on the baby. Fantasies, based on misinformation, can be horrible.

PREPARATION

Before making a decision it is important that the staff understand the fears and illusions the parents may have concerning autopsy. Parents should be approached with respect and compassion. It helps parents to understand that an autopsy or chromosomal study may uncover valuable information as to the cause of the baby's death and the implications for having future children.

Waiting for the results of the autopsy is a stressful time. The results should be reported as soon as possible to the parents by the obstetrician or pediatrician in as clear and concise a manner as possible. Technical, confusing language only deepens their frustration.

"It turned out that the autopsy didn't tell us anything more than anything else. But it was reassuring to look down the list and see all the things that were normal and that everything was within the normal range. It was not reassuring to know that there was really no reason for him to die. But, I think it will make it easier next time because I know that there wasn't anything terribly wrong with him and that we can have a healthy baby."

ARRANGEMENTS

Those who have no choice in their baby's final arrangements will be haunted with the question, "What has happened to my child?" Both fantasies and fears as to what happened to the baby are recurring themes.

Parents must be allowed the right to determine the fate of their babies. Some choose to donate their baby's body to science. Others choose to allow the hospital to arrange for disposition of the body. Some choose to have a full funeral with all the family and friends. Others choose to have a simple service with only family members. Still others decide to cremate the baby and scatter the ashes over the countryside. Some even write their own memorial service. What is done is not as important as the right to have a choice in how to say the final farewells.

Parents who are not allowed a choice, or who are not allowed to be participants in the disposition of their baby may spend the rest of their lives arrested in the early stages of grief, unable to resolve "where the baby is."

The hospital staff can help present options for the final arrangements for the child. They can recommend a chaplain or social worker in the hospital to help the parents discuss the funeral and burial. If the parents experience a miscarriage or early stillbirth, they may, in their shock, think that their only option is to have the hospital take care of their baby's body. Parents may be afraid to ask about what happens to their baby's body. A nurse or doctor should allay these fears and comfort the parents by explaining what is the practice of the hospital.

Where the hospital staff is sensitive to the parents who have lost their baby, there is an evident flexibility in the practices and policies of the hospital for meeting the couple's special needs.

Most bereaved mothers request a private room; nothing is so heartbreaking as to be around mothers whose healthy babies are brought in for nursing, caressing, and cuddling. In fact, many request that they be given a room on another floor.

It is important that the hospital allow the mothers access to their husbands at all times. The greatest fear for the couple is facing the death alone. They need the physical and emotional comfort of each other.

If possible, the mother and father should be offered the services of the hospital chaplain and/or social worker. These professionals have the skills to listen and help parents express their feelings and concerns. If the parents have their own chaplain, priest, or rabbi, he should be contacted and given access at all times. Within reason, family members should also be permitted to visit the parents at any time.

The hospital staff should try to protect the mother and father from insensitive remarks and visits or calls from persons who are not aware of the death and who may upset the parents with their ill-timed visits or words.

Finally, the mother should be allowed to go home as soon as her physical condition permits. Remaining in the hospital reminds her of the baby she will not take home.

> "Probably the A number 1 thing that the hospital did for us was letting Bob stay in the room. We were not charged for that. They left us alone, as much as they could; they recognized our need to be together."

NEED FOR FOLLOW-UP

When the mother goes home she leaves behind the support of her doctors, nurses, and medical staff. But parents are still faced with the hardest questions of all: "How do we answer the insensitive and hurtful comments? How do we get our marriage going again? How do we plan for subsequent pregnancies?"

It is therefore important that the obstetrician schedule an immediate follow-up appointment for both parents. He can then determine how they are handling things, and he may provide new information about the baby's death. The physician may be able to guide the parents in understanding their grief or put them in touch with a support group.

> "I think that the best thing my doctor did to me was say, 'I have made an appointment for you to come see me in one week. Call me if you have something you need to talk about before that. When the autopsy report comes in, let's sit down and talk about it.'"

> "I felt that I got almost zero support. The only thing my doctor said was, 'Call me,' but I didn't think he meant it at all. He never called me back to ask me how things were going, and I didn't see him until my six-week checkup, at which time he didn't seem to want to talk to me about the death."

MESSAGE TO THE STAFF

Some helpful suggestions to the hospital staff:

1. Although it may be the easiest path to take, try not to avoid the parents. They need you to hold their hands and to cry with them.
2. When you are in the room with the parents, talk about the pregnancy, the labor, the delivery, and the baby.
3. Give the parents some privacy. Ask if they would like the door closed. Also, it's important that you screen phone calls and visitors. The more choices parents have, the more they feel in control of a life that has gone out of control.
4. Acknowledge the pain the mother and father are experiencing. Don't say: "I understand how you feel." Rather, state: "This must be the hardest thing you've ever been through."
5. If another delivery is taking place, try to protect the parents from hearing it as much as possible.

6. Don't assume that the parents know things. They need information as to the condition of the baby or why the baby died.
7. The couple needs an opportunity to hold their baby. They need your encouragement to do so, while at the same time they should not feel that you are forcing them.
8. If the baby has abnormalities that are visible, the parents need to know how the baby will look before he/she is brought in. Mention the positive features of the child and do not focus on the abnormalities but be prepared to explain them. Stay with the parents for support.
9. Parents need to know that a photograph or footprint will be kept at the hospital. They need to know that these are available and how to get them when, and if, they so desire.

6

Immediate Feelings

THE IMPORTANCE OF EXPRESSING FEELINGS

Although generally all bereaved parents experience anger, disappointment, confusion, isolation, jealousy, denial, and loss of self-confidence and esteem, these emotions occur with different intensities and at different times for each individual. For parents to hide their thoughts and problems from each other and from other children in the family can be destructive. Silence sometimes leads to emotional and physical breakdown in both the father and the mother. It may even destroy some marriages. Some parents find emotional problems exist not only for the living children but also for future children. It is vital that parents be encouraged to talk and express their feelings.

Of course, communication is essential to any marriage. Partners should be encouraged to talk to each other about the death.

The earlier they can discuss and explore the subject, the better the marriage will be.

Talking with support groups of parents who have also lost babies gives grieving parents an understanding that cannot be gained from anyone else. Just being there and seeing that other parents have survived the experience provides reassurance that "the craziness will end."

> "I didn't need words at that time. I needed to be heard, I needed people to listen to me, to let me talk about the loss and what it meant to me and my family."

> "My husband and I have never really talked about our feelings. I don't think he wants to—and I'm afraid to."

INHIBITING FACTORS TO GRIEVING

Parents find there are three major factors that stand in the way of expressing and working through feelings. One is the different intensity of grief for the mother and father. The second is the cultural conditioning of the father for suppressing his feelings; and the third is the reticence of the hospital staff, family, and friends to provide a nonthreatening and nonjudgmental atmosphere where parents are encouraged to talk about their emotions and to exercise their options.

FEELINGS BETWEEN PARENTS

Many marriages can suffer, at least temporarily, from the frustration and resentment brought on by the difference in intensity of feeling of the two parents. Mothers, having the responsibility of carrying and nurturing the baby, know the unique personalities of their babies for a longer period of time than the fathers. The mother has developed deeper feelings of attachment and so may experience a different level of grief from the father. Parents may sense how diverse their feelings are, and evade the subject of the baby on the pretext that they do not want to bring pain to one another.

CULTURAL CONDITIONING

In our culture women have more experience in openly expressing their feelings, while men are more apt to deny and diminish the importance of their emotions. Men have been taught they must be strong. When the death of his baby occurs, everyone from the hospital staff to the family expects the father to be stable and to support the mother emotionally.

HOSPITAL STAFF

Many parents are afraid to express their feeling to the hospital staff. Some are even apologetic about their sorrow. This may be due to an inability of the doctors and nurses to openly discuss the death of the baby with the parents.

FRIENDS AND FAMILY

Friends and family frequently take special care to talk only about cheerful subjects and are afraid to bring up the death. This avoidance only adds to the pain.

> "I remember at first Paul telling everyone to be strong for me. He told my parents to be strong. No one would cry around me. It made me feel very uncomfortable because it didn't give me the OK to go ahead and cry. I was holding back a lot of the times when I felt like crying. It turns out that they were too. They were all trying to be strong, and I was trying to be strong, and it was really stupid because we should have just been crying and getting it over with together."

THINGS TO SAY TO BEREAVED PARENTS

- It must seem like a bad dream to you and you want to wake up and have it all go away.
- You may be feeling shocked and numb.
- You must be wondering why you are unable to cry. It's a natural first reaction; your tears will come later.
- You must be very sad. It is a terrible thing that has happened to you and your baby.
- We don't know why these things happen; they just do sometimes.

CONFUSION/SHOCK

When birth ends in death, there is confusion. The mother, in disbelief and shock, sees it as a nightmare, willing it to end yet knowing it won't. Mothers who are heavily medicated are in a difficult state of mental turmoil: they are totally out of control, moving in and out of consciousness. The unmedicated mothers are unprepared for what may next happen physically, emotionally, and spiritually. "What has happened?" "Where is my baby?" "What about my husband?" She is confused about what this means to her future. This is not in the order of things. Birth should not end in death.

The father is also disoriented, bouncing between reality and confusion. While everyone is looking to him to be strong he is trying to hold on to reality, but sequences become mixed up and reality moves in and out of focus.

The apparent calm of both parents is a reaction to shock. Assure them they are not insensitive, and gently tell them that they will be able to express their grief in the following days.

> "There is lots of confusion on the part of the mother whose baby has died. A stillbirth, for some reason, presents different states of confusion. When I had a stillbirth, I remember being drugged afterward, so that my confusion had a lot to do with having taken those drugs, and going in and out of confusion."

ANGER

When the hope of pregnancy dies with the baby, both mother and father experience anger. They are angry at their doctor because he promised that with early prenatal care, nutritious diet, and personal care, a healthy baby would be delivered. Parents are angry at the hospital staff because they promised that in the safety of the hospital a safe birth would occur. Parents are angry at themselves for not being able to produce a healthy baby. They are angry at God for letting this senseless thing happen. They are angry when the huge medical bills for a failure of medicine are received, angry with their families and friends and community for their insensitivity, angry because of their isolation, and angry at the dismissal of their grief as trivial.

All parents express anger differently, some quite openly and others more quietly. No matter what its expression, it is real anger that has to be expressed and worked through before grief can be resolved.

> "Then my freakish feeling turned toward hatred toward my doctor. 'That SOB, how could I go on for three months, not growing and he didn't even notice it? He's supposed to be the boy wonder. Where was he?' I used to go bananas. Finally someone said, 'Go and see him, talk to him.' So finally we set up this meeting and we went in and we talked with him and he said, 'Hindsight is always twenty-twenty, and in retrospect, maybe a mistake was made. But I can offer no apologies, because I really believed everything was just fine.'"

"GOING CRAZY"

"I feel as if I am going crazy," is a common and continuous reaction of parents whose babies die. Everything is topsy-turvy, the world has turned around. In place of a crib is a casket. In place of a nursery is an empty room. Nothing prepares parents to think about mortuaries and death certificates. Is the mother going crazy when she still feels her baby moving in her body? Is the father going crazy when he wakens and hears a baby's cry in the nursery? Is their craziness wrecking their marriage when the father is on one crazy level and the mother on another, and they can't even relate?

> "I said to my doctor, 'I think I'm going crazy because I still feel the baby moving inside of me.' He told me 'It's just like when they have to amputate a leg or an arm and the person still feels it's there, and that's going to be with you for a while.' "

DISAPPOINTMENT

Parents are disappointed not only in the death of their baby, but in the death of all the dreams they had for the future. Mothers are disappointed that their bodies have let them down. When parents give birth to a healthy baby, they are surrounded with society's joy and approval. When birth ends in tragedy, grieving parents feel not only their own immense disappointment, they believe they are the source of disappointment for everyone around them.

> "We had planned for this baby, it meant everything to us. Now, our disappointment was overwhelming."

FAILURE

When the death of the infant is announced, parents may believe they are announcing their failure to the world: they have failed in one of the most basic of all missions in life. Their bodies can no longer be relied on. Even their sexuality is challenged. Most of all, parents fear they may never be able to produce a healthy child. They have not only failed as parents but have also failed to fulfill the expectations of society. They have failed their own parents, who were expecting to be grandparents. They have failed their friends and relatives.

> "I was thinking about when we were talking about the feeling of failing as a woman, and I remember when my first child was born, there were so many flowers in my room that you couldn't see out of the window, and my in-laws sent me this big bouquet of roses. When my second baby died, they didn't even acknowledge it, they didn't even send anything to the funeral or anything. It created a tremendous sense of failure."

GUILT

Anger turned inward becomes guilt. When their baby dies the parents spend hours and days going over events and things they had done that might have caused the baby's death. If the death is from genetic abnormalities some parents feel guilty about passing these genetic factors on to other children. If the death is caused by other factors, or if there is no evident reason, the burden of guilt is even greater. These people spend hours searching their backgrounds, looking for an event for which they are being punished. The father may consider his ambivalence or envy during the pregnancy as a cause. The mother may feel anguish about an aspirin she took, a glass of wine, her continuing to work, and any stressful event she experienced during the pregnancy. The couple may feel guilt about having had intercourse toward the end of pregnancy.

"God, I did everything right. The right food, the right classes, the right doctor. It didn't help any. When I was sixteen, I had had an abortion that I didn't tell my husband about. I really feel down deep that the abortion had something to do with my not being able to carry the baby."

"Bob and I are really worried. Our baby died of a recessive genetic defect. Do we have a right to pass it on to our other children? Is the one healthy child we have one day going to look at us and blame us if he and his wife have a defective baby?"

ISOLATION

Parents who produce a healthy baby are surrounded by a community who celebrate the birth. Grandparents, aunts, uncles, sisters, brothers, and friends all come together to congratulate the parents on the precious treasure they have brought into the world. Parents whose baby dies, however, often feel like outcasts who have done something shameful. The grandparents, grieving for their own loss, and other family members may not know how to support the mother and father, and so, they avoid contact. Very few of the parents' friends have faced death, and, not knowing how to meet their needs, may stay away. Pregnant friends avoid contact because of conscious or unconscious fears for themselves and guilt.

"It turns around too, the people you think don't care are often the people who really come through. It's like this beautiful card that I got for Mother's Day. It came from right out of the blue. It wasn't even from a close friend, just someone who knew how I was feeling."

"I really had intense feelings of alone-ness, or sole-ness that nobody else could ever have experienced this kind of thing."

IRRITABILITY

Just at the time when the mother and father need each other as well as outside support, many grieving parents find the least significant thing irritating. Not only have they been through birth, but they have also experienced death. Their tolerance level for handling even the normal stresses of everyday life is dangerously low. It is as if nerves are just below the surface of the skin and they are unable to hold back their reactions. Parents are especially vulnerable to imagined slights, and are unable to handle insensitive or thoughtless remarks from others.

"I don't blame my husband for staying away, all I did was cry and bitch."

JEALOUSY

After the death of their infant, it seems to parents that everywhere they turn there is proof of others' ability to conceive, bear, and give birth to healthy babies. Jealousy is a surprising response. Mothers feel a special jealousy when they are asked to attend a baby shower or when they see other mothers with babies at the supermarket. Attitudes toward pregnant teenagers' unwanted pregnancies are terrible. Sisters and friends who are pregnant and give birth to healthy babies sometimes sense the bereaved parents' attitude and experience guilt themselves.

> "I would stand outside the supermarket and watch other mothers with their babies. And I would feel a great wave of jealousy. I would have to walk away."

PREOCCUPATION

After the baby's death, parents review the events of the birth over and over again. They are preoccupied with each detail that preceded and followed birth and death. Memories plague them for a long time. They may need to hear repeatedly what happened from the medical staff: what went right, what went wrong, what was said. This preoccupation is an important part of the grief work. Although it is painful and exhausting, it helps to make some sense of the baby's death.

> "I was obsessed, I couldn't think of anything but the baby, each moment of the pregnancy, the labor, the delivery, and each minute detail of the death."

> "My friends stopped coming over, and my mother accused me of being preoccupied and morbid. It was driving me crazy—why? why? why?"

7

The Loneliest Grief in the World

The grief of parents over the loss of their baby is the loneliest grief in the world. Usually, when a beloved child dies all of the community surrounds the parents to share their sorrow. Grandparents who loved the child and knew him/her in a special way cry with the parents over their loss. Family and friends share their grief and, because they have children of their own, understand the profound sense of loss.

However, when parents lose a child before or right after birth, no one can share in the terrible sorrow because no one else really knew the baby. People who have not experienced miscarriage, stillbirth, or newborn death cannot fathom the depth of the grief. Statements such as "You can always have another baby"; "It's for the best; the baby was defective anyway"; "God needed another angel"; all demonstrate a lack of understanding and an inability to give the parents the support they need. Instead, these responses make parents feel all the more isolated and without help.

Alone and surrounded by people who cannot support them, the couple naturally turn to each other. The most common expectation is that because they conceived their baby in a mutual act their grief will be shared too. They expect to be strong and to support one another. In reality, while each parent's grief is great, there are differences in origin and/or intensity which may force each of them to go it alone. Perhaps neither parent has the energy or endurance to pick up the pieces and go on with life, let alone be responsible for someone else's life. The terrible toll of their separate grief may be the death of a marriage unless the parents can understand how differently the mother and the father experience grief, how differently they express their feelings, and how different is the time it takes each of them to recover.

PHYSICAL SYMPTOMS OF GRIEF

It is common for parents who have lost their baby to be overwhelmed by a tightness and a choking feeling in their throats. They may feel constantly fatigued, that lifting an arm or a leg is an exhausting effort. The thought of eating is sometimes unbearable. Loss of appetite and an empty feeling in the stomach are common.

Listlessness and an inability to concentrate may persist. Parents may feel as if they had to "do something," but the "something" is vague. These physical symptoms diminish with time, as the intense grief is resolved.

> "I would lie in bed for days; time had no meaning. Days and weeks passed without my knowing."

SLEEPING PROBLEMS

Most bereaved mothers are unprepared for sleeping difficulties. Taking a long walk before bedtime might help the person fall asleep more easily. Avoidance of coffee and caffeine in drinks is a good idea.

> "Bedtime was the absolute worst. I would put it off as long as I could. Then when I finally went to bed I couldn't fall asleep. I would find myself going over the death again and again. After hours of tossing and turning I would only get to sleep to wake up after a nightmare."

> "For months I had the same nightmare, that my baby was alive but needed my help. I would go to get him and I would awake without him. My empty life was crushing."

RESTLESSNESS

Bereaved mothers spend their days in restless, aimless searching for something to do. They may begin one thing and leave it unfinished to begin another. They are unable to start and carry on any organized activity. They find it difficult to concentrate. They may drift in and out of conversations and find themselves stopped in mid-sentence, not remembering what they were talking about.

Although fathers may experience the same feelings of restlessness, they show it in different ways. Many fathers find themselves becoming totally involved in their professions. They approach each task with new fervor, working at such a fast pace so as to forget the baby's death. It is easier to leave the sorrow of the house, the nursery, and the grieving wife, and enter into the no-nonsense world of work. In reality, they may be putting off facing reality and the grief work still before them.

"Right after he was born and died, I threw myself into my work. Part of it was a normal need to do so, and I would have done so under any circumstance, but I'm sure, looking back at it, part of it was just trying to escape, get away, work ten, twelve, fourteen, sixteen hours a day, seven days a week, never home. It wasn't until the early spring that I finally finished the project that I was working on. That's when things really hit me. It was a terrible time."

"I found I couldn't make myself stay in one spot. I moved in and out of rooms, in and out of chairs. I'd pick up something to do and couldn't remember what."

"I had the overwhelming feeling that there was something I must do, but I couldn't find out what."

STAGES OF GRIEF

There is nothing new or startling about the shock, denial, and anger that accompanies tragedy. Depression usually always accompanies the death of a loved one. In the end, most people do resolve the death, make some meaning of it, and move on with their lives.

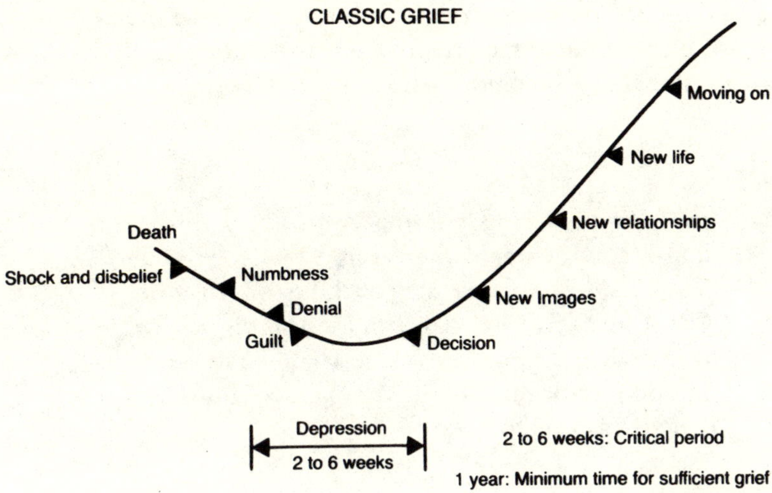

Classic grief after a loss in pregnancy. Reprinted from Perinatology-Neonatology *(Nov.–Dec. 1977), p. 31. Copyright by Barrington Publications, Inc., 825 S. Barrington Avenue, Los Angeles, California 90049.*

Recent work by Elizabeth Kübler-Ross and others has made important contributions to grief work by recognizing a pattern in these reactions. They have outlined the normal and natural stages most people go through to regain peace of mind after a loved one dies. These stages of shock, denial, bargaining and guilt, anger, depression, and acceptance serve as a framework to help parents and people who wish to help them accept the normality of their feelings, understand the importance of expressing the feelings they are experiencing, and gain hope that the pain does diminish, and that they can and will survive the experience. But every person grieves differently: some spend more time in bargaining or in anger, some do not go through every stage. What is important is that, in time, each person moves on and does not remain locked in one stage. A parent who cannot move on from anger or depression, for example, should seek professional psychological help.

> "A lot of the books were telling me about the stages of grief. And I kept wondering 'Am I doing this right?' It almost sounded as if there was a real format and you could just wake up and say 'Well, I'm out of shock now.' And I just thought, 'Am I doing this right?' But then again, when I'd go to group or whatever, it was just like 'I'm doing it right.' There's no pattern, there's nothing that you can really follow."

HOW LONG DOES IT TAKE?

There is no specific length of time in which grief is resolved or each phase passed through. The stages can overlap, with the mother or father being depressed while at the same time angry. The stages may recur at any time with guilt or depression sweeping over the parent at unexpected moments. Their order and degree of intensity may vary for every parent's experience. A mother who has experienced miscarriage may have greater feelings of guilt. A mother who experienced stillbirth may experience greater feelings of depression. A mother who loses a newborn may have greater feelings of anger. The grieving process may take from six to twenty-four months. But the bereaved mother and father lose track of days and weeks and months, and the first year may be perceived as lost in time. Events of the death remain vivid, and it may seem as if they took place only yesterday.

Total acceptance or resolution of the grief may never take place completely. There will be times, even years later, that an event, a song, a special day will bring back the grief; but it is a grief that is not so overwhelming and intense. The grief is now manageable, and has diminished in intensity.

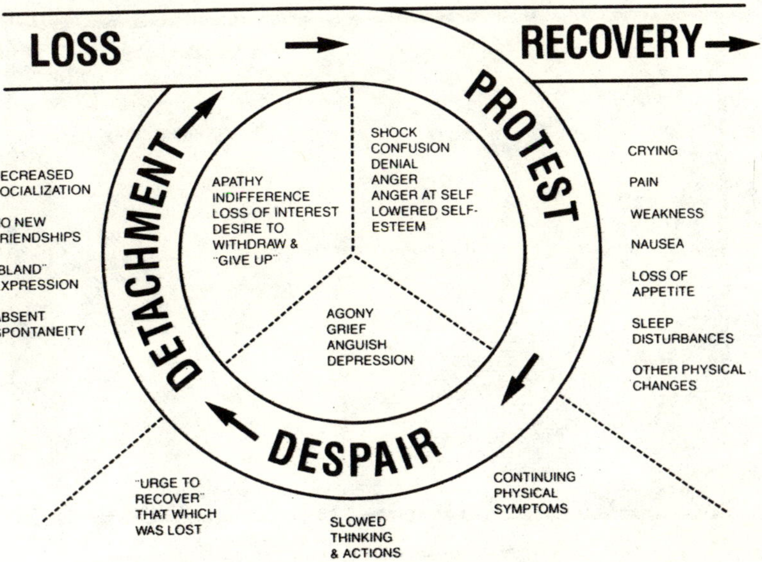

SHOCK AND DENIAL

The first stage of most parents' grief is shock, disbelief, and denial. The death is just too sudden and the loss too great to comprehend. Shock delays its impact and gives the parent time to gather his/her resources and to absorb the depth of the tragedy. Numbness and not being able to respond or cry are common indications of shock. At no other time does the parent feel so much alone.

This is the time when the medical staff can offer important support. They should not tranquilize or medicate the mother in an effort to spare her pain. A groggy, medicated mother will have a harder time resolving her grief than one who is unmedicated. They should understand that the seeming calm of the parents is a shock reaction. Assuring the parents that they are not insensitive, that their grief will be expressed in the fol-

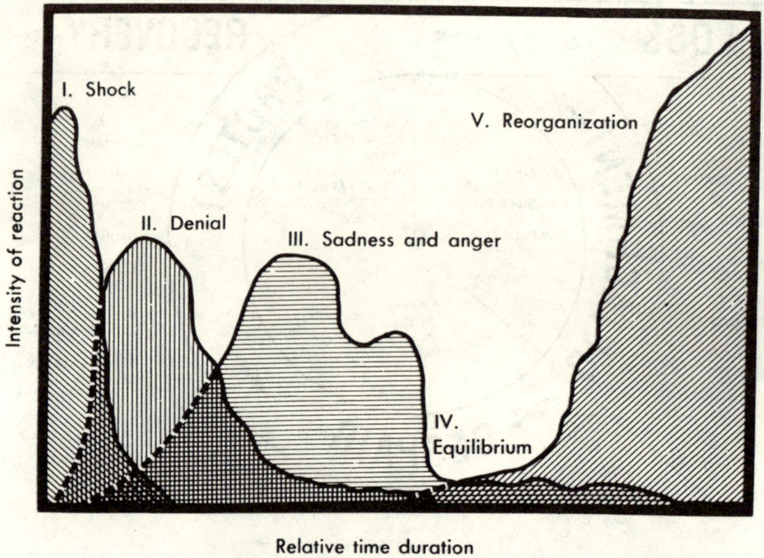

Hypothetical model of the sequence of normal parental reactions to the birth of a child with congenital malformations. From D. Drotar, A. Baskiewicz, N. Irvin, J. H. Kennell, and M. H. Klaus, Pediatrics *56, no. 5 (Nov. 1975), pp. 710–717, fig. 1. Copyright © 1975 by American Academy of Pediatrics.*

lowing days will greatly aid them. In addition, seeing, holding, touching, and saying good-bye to the baby can help the parents accept the reality of the death.

> "I can remember walking around just feeling totally like a zombie, thinking, 'What's going on? What's happening?' Almost as if I were standing there looking at myself and saying, 'This isn't happening to me, it couldn't be happening to me.' It was a total denial of reality."

"For the next couple of days I tried to deal with it on a realistic level. But I kept thinking, 'This couldn't have happened.' I was sure that if I blinked only two minutes would have passed and it would be just a bad dream."

"I think at that point I was so numb that leaving the hospital without the baby really didn't hit me. I was still drugged up a little bit. If I had stayed around a couple of days and recovered, I would have been a lot more devastated walking out that front door without a bundle in my arms. It really didn't hit me until a couple of days later."

SUGGESTED THINGS TO SAY

- It must seem like a bad dream to you. You must want to wake up and have it all go away.
- It is natural for you to be shocked and numb. This doesn't mean you don't care and that you won't grieve later.
- You must be very sad, it is a terrible thing that has happened to you and your baby. I wish it weren't true, but it is.

EMOTIONAL SYMPTOMS

BARGAINING AND GUILT

Bargaining is a return to childhood, when we believed we could strike a deal with God. "If I only do this, I can make my baby live." It's a desperate move to retain some control over a life that has gone out of control.

Guilt can be one of the strongest and longest-lasting emotions. When the bargains don't work, the anger can turn inward to guilt. The parents blame themselves for the tragedy and wonder what they did to cause it.

The greatest help the couple can receive is for others to recognize their guilt feelings and assure them it is normal to blame themselves and feel they are being punished.

"Unfortunately, we had had intercourse the night before the baby died. When I went into early labor the next day and the baby was too small to live, we both couldn't help blaming ourselves for causing premature labor. Our doctor assured us that the baby died for other reasons, but it has still affected our sex life. The spark has gone from our marriage and I don't think it will ever be the same again."

SUGGESTED THINGS TO SAY

- I know you must be feeling guilty for your baby's death. It's hard not to feel that it is your fault. It's difficult to accept that there is no accountable reason for your baby's death. But sometimes these things are out of our control.
- It's common to try to find reasons for your baby's death. It all seems so futile and out of control.
- It sounds as if you think your smoking caused your baby's death. We know that, although smoking is not good for a baby, your baby died for other reasons and smoking was not a part of it.
- I know you would do anything to give your baby a healthy life again, and we would too. We will do everything to support you and your baby, but it looks as if your baby's problems are too great for his or her survival.

ANGER

As parents begin to recognize the reality of the baby's death, most experience overwhelming anger at the senselessness and futility of the death, at themselves for failing at birth, at the baby for leaving them, at each other, at the doctor, at friends and family for not being able to help, and even at God for allowing this to happen.

It is important to understand that anger is one step toward final acceptance of the baby's death. It is vital to be able to express anger, envy, resentment, and rage, to acknowledge it, and to realize that these are common and normal reactions to the tragedy.

Parents who are unable to express their anger may experience a greater and longer depression than those who can. The doctor and the nurses who surround the grieving couple may find it difficult to support the parents because they too have suffered a loss. They too may have feelings of anger and helplessness. It is important that the staff work to overcome this by admitting their own anger and even sharing it with the parents.

> "The thing I was really angry at, and I'm still angry at, is that I was the perfect case. I did everything so right. I had the perfect blood pressure, the perfect urine sample. I ate right, I even left the room if someone smoked. I did everything right. It didn't make any difference. I'm still angry when I see all these people who smoke and drink and still put out healthy babies with no effort at all. It scares me, because I think next time all I can do is do everything perfect like I did the last time, and just cross my fingers and hope that this time I'm lucky. But it still comes back to: Why me when I did everything so right?"

> "I was angry at my mother. I was angry at my father. I was angry at my brothers, sister-in-law, at my friend in New York who drank and smoked. I went through such unbelievable anger. I was angry at the entire medical profession, not just my doctor. I went through the real, hair-raising, almost bottle-throwing, ripping, screaming, crying, hysterical anger. The day I got home from the genetics clinic, I wanted to go out and stomp on the baby's grave I was so angry. I was hysterical."

SUGGESTED THINGS TO SAY

- It is natural to feel anger and hostility toward everyone and everything that had to do with your baby's death. I feel angry too.
- You must be very angry that your baby has suffered, and you can do nothing about it.
- It is normal and reasonable to be angry and resentful when you have lost your baby, and others have live and healthy babies.
- It must be hard to find the words to express your anger, helplessness, and frustration.
- It is important that you allow yourself to express your anger and rage no matter how much others try to discourage you.
- You have lost your baby and you have a right to be angry and frustrated.

DEPRESSION

Once parents have passed through shock, denial, and anger, most will settle into a period that is heavy with great sadness and depression. Their lives have lost meaning, and it is more than they can do to get up every morning to face their empty arms, empty nursery, empty future. Many go through a period of questioning the meaning of life and death. There can be a terrible feeling of pain, a deep sense of despair, and an overwhelming emptiness.

Parents now need someone who is with them physically, emotionally, and spiritually. They do not need cheering up. In fact, at this stage words are probably the last thing they need. What they do need is someone to listen to their pain.

"I forgot to eat. When someone would remind me to eat, I couldn't taste the food and it stayed like a lump in my throat."

"There wasn't anything that didn't remind me of the baby I did not have. Every newspaper or magazine I picked up was full of happy babies and parents. Everyone I had ever known was pregnant or had a new baby."

"My depression was overwhelming. I couldn't get up to answer the door, I wouldn't answer the phone. I couldn't even find the energy to keep myself clean. I could only go over again and again the senselessness of the death."

"I didn't want to be around anybody. I threw myself into my work fourteen hours a day, scrambling to keep ahead of the depression. I now know that I was only putting it off for another time."

SUGGESTED THINGS TO SAY

- **It's normal to be depressed when you have lost one of your most precious treasures.**
- **It must be painful to see your nursery empty of all your dreams.**
- **You have lost your baby and have a right to be depressed.**

ACCEPTANCE

After working through the feelings of denial, anger, guilt, and depression, bereaved parents finally come to the stage where they accept the fact of the death. The hurt and empty space are still there and always will be, but they can laugh and make plans again. They can now talk calmly about the life and death of the baby and what he/she meant to their lives.

Some parents find new meaning in religion, some in an outside activity, some in a job. Many find new meaning in joining or beginning a support group for parents to give them the support they need and in finding new friends.

As they come through the grief, the parents grow and change in many ways. Their relationships and their ability to cope have been tested, and they have survived. They find new strengths, and, as the pain subsides, they begin to take up their lives again.

"I'm not really sure how we put it back together. Through all the tears of grieving I realized that I had survived a year; our marriage had survived. I decided to go to a part-time job. I had friends and I was okay."

"I finally accepted the death when I accepted the risk to become pregnant again and get on with my life. I shall never forget my baby—but now I can accept my new child for himself and not as a replacement in my life."

SHADOW GRIEF

Bereaved parents can be surprised by grief at times when they are totally unprepared for it. It may appear at an invitation to a friend's baby shower, to a christening. Dates such as the baby's first birthday or the anniversary of his/her death are especially difficult. Christmas, Thanksgiving, and other family holidays always remind parents of their baby and how it might have been if he or she had lived.

> "Every anniversary of my baby's death takes me by surprise. I think I'm not going to remember it and then when the day is on me I go into a deep depression, even if I don't know consciously what the day is."

> "Christmas reminds me of the empty place that will never be filled by the baby we lost. It's not a deep pain, but a kind of lonely ache."

> "Every anniversary my husband sends me three red roses for our three living children and one white rose for the baby who has died."

WHEN TO SEEK PROFESSIONAL HELP

Here are some general guidelines to determine when parents may be in need of professional help.

1. Persistence of denial: A mother or father who remains in the denial stage may need counseling. Keeping the nursery exactly as it was and not putting away the baby's clothes or toys are signs of denial.

2. Persistence in anger or guilt: Parents who cannot move on from the rage they first felt are also having difficulties. They are still paralyzed by their anger or desire for revenge toward their doctor, hospital, staff, or themselves.

3. Persistence of depression: Sometimes a mother or father remains in a deep depression that does not allow her/him to get on with life. Persistent sleep difficulties, loss of appetite, irritability, crying, fatigue, intense feelings of guilt, anger, blame, or worthlessness many weeks after the death are indicators of difficulties in resolving grief.

4. Inability to function: A mother or father whose inner feelings prevent her/him from returning to the outside world to function and work in a healthy way needs help with this problem.

5. Self-destructive thoughts or behavior require immediate attention.

8

What Happens Next? At Home

PHYSICAL RECOVERY

The six weeks after birth is a special period called postpartum. During this period the woman deals with her body as she recovers from the pregnancy, labor, and delivery. It is traditionally a difficult time for women who bring their healthy babies home with them. For a mother who has lost her baby, it can be a nightmare. Not only is she experiencing grief from the death of her child, but she must also contend with the discomfort of the stitches of an episiotomy, vaginal bleeding, breasts filled with useless milk, and changing hormones. When she leaves the hospital she should be given instructions to help her deal with these discomforts.

STITCHES

If, during birth, an episiotomy (a surgical cut between the vagina and rectum to make more room for the baby's delivery) was performed, the mother will have stitches to repair the cut. There may be pain or itching as the stitches are absorbed or drop out during the healing process. Using a heat lamp or taking sitz baths may reduce that pain. Applying an ice pack will reduce swelling. If the pain is severe, the mother should tell the doctor. Complete, firm healing of the episiotomy may take several weeks.

VAGINAL BLEEDING

The mother will be dealing with a vaginal discharge called lochia. Lochia comes from the site where the placenta detached from the wall of the uterus. It is usually bright red the first day and by the third day it decreases in flow and becomes lighter in color. By the tenth day the discharge is often pale yellow and sticky or watery. If at any time the mother uses more than two pads in one hour, or the discharge has a foul smell, or turns to bright red she should contact her doctor immediately, since she might have an infection.

AFTERPAINS

Contractions clamp down on the open uterine blood vessels after birth and help the uterus return to its normal condition. These contractions, often called afterpains, are less intense with the first baby and more intense with subsequent births. They may continue for several days and occasionally are severe enough to require medication. Concentration on deep breathing and relaxation may help the mother ease her discomfort.

SWOLLEN BREASTS

Many mothers who experience a late miscarriage, stillbirth, or newborn death are horrified to find that their breasts, unaware of the death, continue in their mission to feed the baby. The accompanying pain of engorgement reminds her that there is no baby to give her relief. Ice packs help to reduce the swelling and a tight bra or binder helps to keep the milk supply low. An aspirin may relieve the pain. The mother should be instructed not to express the milk because that only encourages more milk production.

POSTPARTUM BLUES

Even a mother who has a healthy baby may experience postpartum blues. The tremendous drop in hormonal levels following the birth is responsible for emotional fluctuations. It's common for all new mothers to experience a mild irritability and depression, which usually goes away. However, when the grieving mother experiences these hormonal drops her emotional fluctuations and depression are compounded. She has very little reserve with which to cope, and her depression is profound. She feels out of control, irritated with everything, and unable to cope with the enormous tragedy that has fallen into her life.

FATIGUE

Every new mother is surprised by the unexpected amount of fatigue and exhaustion she experiences for the first few weeks. The bereaved mother finds her energy sources depleted. Her fatigue is increased by the additional energy it takes to grieve for her baby and she is overwhelmed.

COMPLICATIONS

Because of the overwhelming stress a bereaved mother has experienced, she may be more susceptible to complications in her postpartum recovery. It is important that she be aware of the symptoms that could signal problems. Both she and her husband should be given instructions to call the doctor if she experiences any of the following:

Excessive fatigue
Fever or chills
Abdominal cramps or tenderness
Bleeding that persists, becomes excessive, bright red, or has a foul smell
Tenderness or redness in the calves of her legs
Sore, warm, or inflamed areas in her breasts
Burning sensations when she urinates
Severe or prolonged depression

THE FIRST POSTPARTUM CHECKUP

When the first postpartum checkup is due, the mother may dread returning to her doctor's office. She knows the waiting room is full of pregnant mothers or new mothers who have brought in their healthy babies all dressed in ruffles and bows. How can she stand those horrible reminders? Yet, she is anxious to talk with her doctor about some questions.

Many mothers call the office in advance, and request to be allowed to wait someplace more private. Often, this can be especially helpful because many times the office nurse and staff don't realize the patient has lost her baby. The mother should go with her husband or a family member for more support. Before the visit it is important to list all the questions and concerns.

Once at the doctor's office, it is vital that the parents understand as much about the death as possible. The doctor should discuss how this death might affect any future pregnancies, and any treatment or diagnostic testing that could be of help. If the parents take notes they can go over the information again and again. If the doctor hands out literature or books, it helps in further understanding. Some parents can talk openly and freely with their doctor about depression and their marriage. Advice on participating in a local support group or finding professional help is also appropriate.

> "My doctor's nurse didn't even know about the death and asked me what I had, a boy or girl. I broke into tears and ran out. My husband had to bring me back."

> "My doctor had me come in the first visit after lunch. He didn't let me wait and I really appreciated that. I'll always love him because he didn't only care about my physical recovery, but he looked me in the eye and asked me how was I *really* doing. And I know he wanted to hear my answer no matter how bad it was."

SOME IMPORTANT QUESTIONS FOR THE DOCTOR TO ASK

- How are you feeling physically? Are you having any problems?
- Are you especially tired? Do you have trouble sleeping?
- What questions do you have about your baby?
- How are you feeling emotionally? How is your husband feeling?
- How is your marriage going? Are you having any problems?
- Do you have questions about other pregnancies?
- Have you had any experiences with friends or family that have disturbed you?
- How do you feel about the choices you made in the hospital? Have you any second thoughts?
- Do you need more information about the death? Does your husband need information?
- Can I give you information on support groups concerned with infant death?

BREAKING THE NEWS TO OTHERS

"I felt like I was the only one it had ever happened to. I wondered: How am I ever going to explain this to anybody? I couldn't believe that anyone could understand."

"I didn't even know how to explain it to people. I just called up our friends and said, 'Well, we were just at the end of labor and our baby died.' I didn't hem or haw and say it was a stillbirth, or we lost the baby. I didn't know any other way to explain it, other than this is where we were, and there was no heartbeat, and the baby just died."

Let people know in as straightforward and simple a way as possible.

- Our baby died last night and I need you now more than ever.
- Something went wrong at the birth and our baby wasn't strong enough to survive.
- I know you shared in our excitement during the pregnancy and would want to share with us in our sadness.
- It seems as if the umbilical cord was compressed and couldn't get oxygen to our baby.
- This is as hard for you to hear as it is for me to say, but our baby was born too early and just didn't have the strength to live.

TELLING THE CHILDREN AT HOME

Although all children will be affected by the death of an infant sibling, each will express him- or herself differently. One may whine and be difficult; another may show aggressive or destructive behavior; some may become angry or withdrawn; others may be fearful or clinging.

Children who are not given information about the baby's death sense that the topic cannot be discussed. They become confused or fearful. Children can create fantasies that are more frightening than reality. No matter what their age, children react more healthily if they are given clear, simple explanations that are appropriate for their ages. They need a real understanding of what has happened, and they need to make sense out of it in their own words.

EXPRESSING FEELINGS

The children are grieving too, and it is just as important that they be given an environment where they can express and work out their feelings as it is for the parents. If the parents are open in expressing grief and feelings, the children will feel safe in doing the same.

FEAR

Death is frightening to all children no matter what age. It makes them realize how vulnerable they are. Children need the assurance that just because the baby died, their lives are not in danger. The best way to tell them what caused the baby's death is in clear, concise, and simple language. If the cause of death is unknown it is important to reassure them that although the baby was not big enough, or healthy enough, or strong enough to survive on his/her own, the living child is indeed strong and healthy and need not fear death.

LONELINESS

Just as the baby's death makes the parents feel lonely and isolated, so it is with the children. It is important to stay close and give them a feeling of belonging and safeness. Because of their vulnerability children need special protection. The most important thing is to just be there, touching, holding, and imparting love to them.

REASSURANCE

A bereaved family will be shaken; life will seem crazy for all members. Each child in the family wonders about his or her place. It is important to find the energy somehow to reassure the children that each is an important, loved, and special member of the family.

> "My son was only two and a half at the time, but I sometimes think he had a sixth sense about what happened. He came in and he crawled up in my lap and he said, 'Oh, Mama, I love you.' I think the one thing that pulled me through those times was every time I got absolutely miserable I would just look at this kid and say, 'Oh God, at least I've got you.'"

> "We wanted to spare our daughter the news of the death—we thought she was too young to understand. But I could tell from her change in behavior—she got so whiny and difficult when she knew something was going on. I never did face it with her, I didn't have the strength then and I don't want to bring it up now. But if I had it to do over, I would have included her in our grief."

> "Our little boy got so he wouldn't let me out of his sight. He was sure that something was going to happen to me, or to his father. He began to have nightmares. These lasted about twelve months and then went away. I knew he couldn't express his grief with words, and I sometimes wonder what those nightmares were about."

FACING PEOPLE

Although everyone wants to be helpful, not everyone is able to say and do the things that can help. On the contrary, insensitive things are said and done that only intensify the parents' anger, frustration, and resentment. Those parents who are prepared in advance for some of these thoughtless comments are better able to respond. Those who are not may become confused and alarmed when confronted.

Some of the insensitive comments that a mother or father who has lost a baby may hear are:

- You really are lucky—that's just nature's way of getting rid of defective babies.
- You are young—you can have lots more babies.
- Isn't it about time that you have gotten yourself together and moved on with your life?
- Well, it's fortunate that you really didn't get to know your baby before it died.
- God needed another angel. Your baby is happy in heaven.
- Why don't you get busy and forget your grief? Join clubs, have your hair done—do anything besides sitting here and feeling sorry for yourself.

The first thing grieving parents must learn is that no matter what anyone says they have a right to grieve, to be angry, depressed, and resentful. These feelings are not only normal but are an important part of working through the grief.

The second thing to be learned is that all parents have a right to love their babies. Anyone who diminishes the intensity of love does not comprehend the death.

The third thing to learn is that parents have the right to remember that the baby is a unique and precious individual who can never be replaced by any other human being. The baby has a place in the family, and, although he or she died in infancy, he or she will always be alive in the parents' memories. Every birthday, Christmas, holiday, and anniversary of his/her death, the parents will remember and wonder.

"I would just give up on some people and tell my husband to tell them that I wasn't at home."

"Some people would never learn, but I learned to live without them and their insensitive remarks."

FUNERAL ARRANGEMENTS

The last rights and responsibilities of parents are to make final arrangements for the baby. Many times, the plans made help parents feel they have some control. The smallest choices made over the service, the clothes, and the site give comfort. Sometimes well-meaning people take over and make arrangements; later, the parents often suffer over their lost control.

The father, assuming the responsibility in his efforts to be strong and save the mother from pain, may make all the funeral arrangements without consulting her. Not only does this responsibility of making arrangements fall on him at a time when his own grief is overwhelming, but the unconsulted mother may feel cheated that she was not allowed to be part of the decision making.

Our society has spent billions of dollars avoiding pain and death. When a baby's death confronts us there are few traditional channels to turn to. If the parents have a funeral for the baby it may help bring the family and community together to provide support. A funeral provides a place for caring persons to express their feelings of sorrow and helps parents face the reality of the death and move on in their grief work, as well as establishing the existence of the child.

If the mother is hospitalized at the time of the funeral, she can still be included in the plans. Photographs can be taken and a tape of the service can even be made for her. She can visit the baby's grave site after she leaves the hospital.

Those parents who choose not to have a funeral, but to have

the hospital take care of the baby, have other options. One of the most satisfying is to have a memorial service, either a small private service (just the parents, or including family and friends). Some parents plant a tree or a flower to honor the memory of their baby.

"Bob and I had Stephan cremated. There was a special place for us up in the mountains. We went up there with the ashes and scattered them in this one spot. And we had a whole bunch of flowers with us, out of which I saved a single yellow rose. We did a lot of crying, and we said things: how we felt about him, and about each other at that time."

"We had a funeral for Juliana. When the day arrived it wasn't as hard as I thought it would be. Our priest was fantastic and the talk he gave was important because all of our closest friends and family were all there and they all got to share in this. My friend said that even though the casket was closed just being there and seeing the burial, Juliana became a person in all of their eyes."

"We didn't have a church and we had never had to make funeral arrangements before. So we invited thirty or forty of our closest friends to our house. We talked a little about our baby after everybody got there. They were so wonderful and supportive that it became more like a wake. When everybody left it made me feel so good to be surrounded by all these people who care. Bringing them together in a group allowed them to talk about their feelings. It eased a lot of tension and they are not going to have to think: Oh, God, what am I going to say to her now?"

PUTTING AWAY THE NURSERY

The first room that the mother is drawn to as she returns home is the nursery. In it are all of the precious clothes, toys, and articles she collected in preparation for her baby's homecoming. As she touches each thing, her pain and feelings of failure are renewed.

Although putting away the nursery is one of the most painful and difficult acts, it is also a way to help mourn the loss and grasp the final reality of the death. There is no one "right" way to handle the nursery. Both parents need to make the decision of how the various belongings should be handled.

Some parents are grateful when mothers or friends offer to pack away the toys, clothes, and other treasures for another time. Others need to do this for themselves.

> "I think the thing I dreaded most was facing the nursery. I was drawn to it like a magnet. When I saw all the sweet toys and clothes that we had gathered for our baby, the full realization of our baby's death hit me for the first time."

> "I couldn't believe it. They took everything away without even asking me. I was numb at first and didn't say anything. But I get furious every time I think about going into that nursery and seeing it bare. I know they meant well, but that was the last thing I could do for my baby."

FINANCIAL PROBLEMS

Along with the death, parents are often overwhelmed with bills: bills from the hospital, the obstetrician, the attending staff, doctors never seen or heard of. There is no baby, only bills. It is a strange irony that leaves a bitter taste. The stress of such financial burdens adds to the bitterness. The worry about money, and the inability to talk about it to anyone, only adds more problems in resolving the baby's death.

> "We had nothing—no baby and now no money. The arguments became endless. It's been harder on our marriage than our baby's death."

9

Stress on the Marriage

EFFECTS ON THE MARRIAGE

Most couples experience new stresses in their marriage after the death of their baby. No matter what the relationship was before the death, many changes occur after the loss. Usually both parents and society assume the loss will bring the parents together, and while sometimes this is the case, more often it is not.

The way each person grieves is dependent on many factors such as past experiences with grief, capacity to handle stress, ability to express feelings, and communication skills. Husbands and wives find themselves grieving separately. When grieving does not fit the expectations of the partner, frustration and resentment are sure to arise. Even the closest of couples sometimes find that they can provide only limited support to one another.

FACTORS PREVENTING CONFLICT BETWEEN HUSBAND AND WIFE

- Sharing the pregnancy. When a couple has shared the pregnancy, such as by attending childbirth classes, they will be better able to share the loss

- Sharing the loss. Being together at the initial time of loss makes the death itself less likely to become a source of conflict in the marriage.
- Being informed. Finding out about the causes of death and about further implications and the hope for future pregnancies will help the couple resume their lives.
- Communicating. Sharing their feelings and also admitting to the differences in the intensity of their feelings will help bring a couple closer together in their tragedy rather than driving them apart.

PREDICTOR OF OUTCOMES OF GRIEF ON THE MARRIAGE*

POSITIVE OUTCOMES	NEGATIVE OUTCOMES
Pregnancy planned	Pregnancy unplanned
Both involved in pregnancy	Father detached from pregnancy
Both informed on childbirth	One or both uninformed on childbirth
Both freely express emotions	One or both unfree to express emotion
Both grieve together	Each grieves separately
Each finds time to be alone	Find little time to be alone
Both overcome societal dictates	One or both submit to societal dictates
Both look for positive aspects	One or both dwell on negative aspects
Both communicate	One or both do not communicate
Each empathetic with other's feelings	One or both self-centered
Both have strong outside support system	Both have little support

*Based on Larry G. Peppers and Ronald J. Knapp, *Motherhood and Mourning: Perinatal Death* (New York: Praeger Publishing, 1980), p. 76.

POSTPARTUM—PULLING TOGETHER

During the postpartum period immediately following the death, the couple gives the appearance of being drawn closer together. The couple is often pulled together by its feeling of isolation from the outside world, but in some instances the couple appears to be close simply because society expects that kind of response.

During this early period both parents are in a confused state of shock. The loss of the baby is usually the first encounter with death. The couple is unsure how to act, what to say. So, in their mutual confusion the mother and father come together, clinging to one another, trying their best to give solace to each other. Yet, neither has the experience or the strength to give the other what is needed.

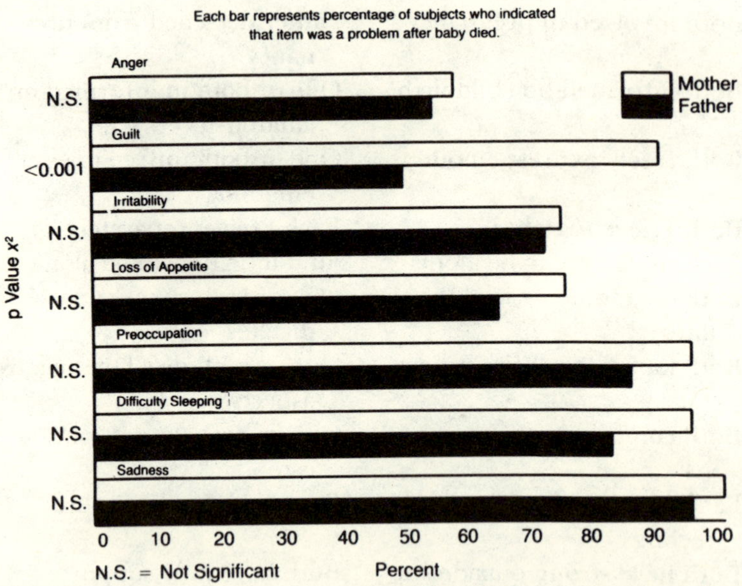

Frequency and comparison of parent grief responses. From J. Cullberg, "Mental Reactions of Women to Perinatal Death," Psychosomatic Medicine in Obstetrics and Gynaecology, *3rd International Congress, London 1971 (Basel: S. Karger AG, 1972), p. 326.*

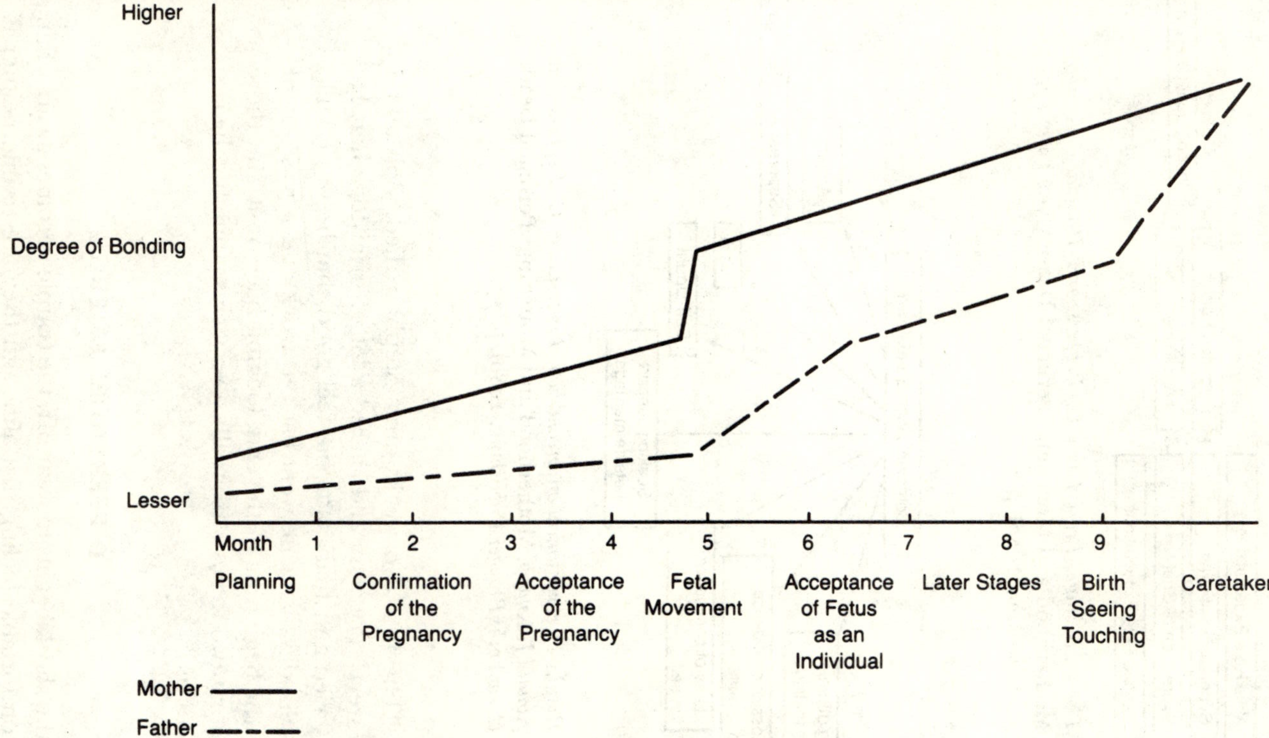

Incongruent bonding of mothers and fathers. From Larry G. Peppers and Ronald J. Knapp, Motherhood and Mourning: Perinatal Death *(New York: Praeger Publishing, 1980), p. 64.*

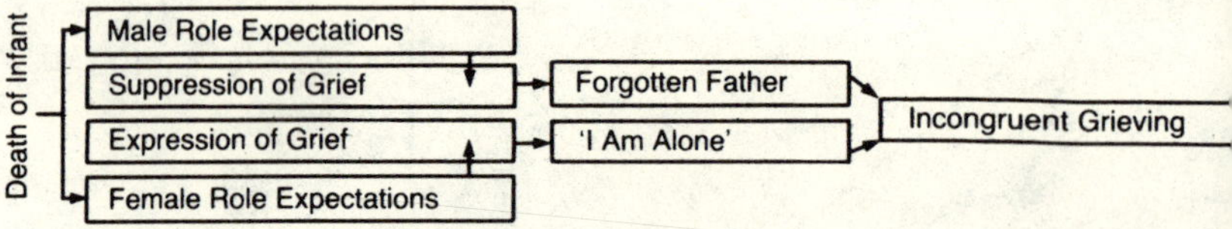

The crisis stage. From Larry G. Peppers and Ronald J. Knapp, Motherhood and Mourning: Perinatal Death *(New York: Praeger Publishing, 1980), p. 78.*

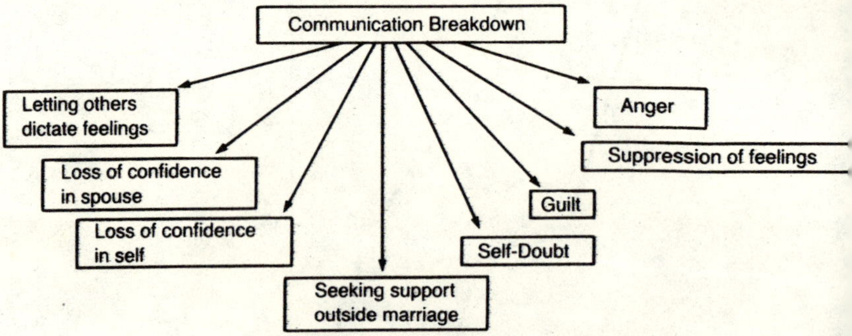

Results of communication breakdown. From Larry G. Peppers and Ronald J. Knapp, Motherhood and Mourning: Perinatal Death *(New York: Praeger Publishing, 1980), p. 77.*

"The first two weeks after Stephan died, Bob and I were very close and shared a lot of grief together. He cried and that made me feel good that he was crying. Six days later he went back to work and it was sort of the beginning of the end, looking back on it. But those first two weeks were really a very close time for the two of us."

DIFFERENCES EMERGE

As the shock begins to wear off, the couple becomes aware of an uncomfortable feeling that although they are trying, neither is meeting the other partner's needs. Differences begin to emerge. Most usually the mother feels that the father cannot comprehend the depth of her grief and resents the father's seeming shallowness. The father begins to experience some frustration with the endurance and depth of the mother's grief. Always hanging over them is a cloud of unspoken blame, guilt, and suspicion that the death was caused through some negligence or defect in either or both of the parents. The differences in grieving and the unrealistic expectations on both sides begin to build a wall between the parents. Each is too overwhelmed with anger and confusion to comprehend that the partner might be grieving in a different way. They concentrate on their differences instead of accepting that there is no one right way to grieve.

"By the end of the first four weeks, we were not getting along at all. The tension of waiting for the genetic report, which may have information that would preclude us from having more children, was great. So we were not only grieving for Stephan, but we were grieving for the possibility of not having children again. And it was just really blowing up for us."

"In the very beginning we were closer than ever. Then we hit a point about two months afterward when I felt that Jim wasn't feeling the death as deeply as I was. He felt that because the genetic results were in our favor we should be grateful because we didn't have to worry about hereditary problems. I went through a period of two or three weeks when I think I almost hated him. He kept saying 'Oh, this is great, we can still have another baby.' And I hated him for not understanding."

COMMUNICATION BREAKDOWN

Tensions are bound to occur between couples who have lost their baby, and failure to communicate is one of the most serious obstacles faced in resolving these tensions. In fact, researchers have observed that some couples do not ever talk about the loss with one another. This inability to express feelings takes its toll on both the father and the mother.

Some fathers try to be cheerful to make the mothers feel better. They are concerned that if they show their grief it will be worse for the mothers. The mothers often see this as a sign of indifference over the death of the baby.

As long as the couple is unable to express their feelings to one another, there may remain a block in the marriage.

> "It just came to a point where we weren't communicating at all, and when we were it was just a lot of fighting. I knew that I was being selfish, but I really didn't care. I just felt like I wanted to be left alone. I wanted to grieve, to cry, to feel sorry for myself, to feel angry. He felt it was time that we begin to go out. I was experiencing these feelings so strongly that I just couldn't make any pretense of going and having dinner with somebody and making conversation about everyday things. I began to feel really angry with him, and he began doing things without me and making excuses to our friends. I felt no guilt about it at all—but things were sure breaking up."

THE CHASM GROWS

Each parent, in trying to cope with grief, finds less and less energy to help the other. The result is disappointment in not being able to support each other. Then the normal responses of anger, guilt, and blaming become attached to issues other than the death. Any trouble experienced by the couple before the death—sex, money, religion, or in-law problems—surfaces and becomes an issue to conceal the real one—guilt for the death of the baby.

If the baby has died for genetic reasons, it becomes even harder to keep the guilt and blame from breaking up a marriage. Resentment and frustration make it hard for the couple to help each other. As the tension mounts, professional family therapy is often needed.

"In the meantime our relationship was deteriorating at a fast rate. When people would ask me how I was doing I would always say, 'Oh, everything is just wonderful.' It really wasn't, but I was playing a game. I still had a need to talk about our baby with my husband. The anticipation of the genetics conference and the anticipation of another baby paralyzed both of us."

"I was getting tired of my wife's grieving. She stayed at home, didn't keep the house, she let herself go, and didn't seem to care about anything. I tried to help cheer her up, but nothing I did seemed to make any difference. I finally had to get out of the house and start doing things on my own. I did begin to wonder when this was going to stop and when we were going to get our life back together—if ever."

"I threw myself into my work. I hadn't gotten much work done during the last six weeks, and so now I felt I had to get cracking on it. I felt so much pressure that I worked from morning to night—I hardly got home. I know now it was just an escape mechanism. I had to take my mind off of the death, just forget about it. Nancy and I drew further and further apart. It seemed as if the chasm was too great to bridge at times."

OPENING COMMUNICATIONS

Open communications can only take place when each parent realizes that the other has a different view of the birth and death, and that each has his or her own way and time frame in which to grieve. Talking about the baby is a way of sharing the loss and reassuring each other that the baby did exist and is part of the family. Most mothers simply want to express their feelings and are not asking for help when the subject comes up repeatedly. Many times fathers interpret the mother's sadness as a cry for help, but the father must realistically accept that there are just some things neither can do for the other. Listening is the key.

"I finally reached a point where I realized that I couldn't go on like this and that my marriage would end in ruins if I didn't make some effort. I had learned a long time ago that if I step outside myself a little bit I'm surprised how much better I feel if I have a good laugh, or watch a good movie. So accidentally I fell into that, and I did begin to feel better. My husband and I began to talk more, and eventually laugh together again."

"One evening I got very upset and told my husband 'You just have to tell me how you are feeling, because I don't think you really care anymore. I think that you have put this behind you and if you have I will hate you forever.' And he said, 'I didn't realize you were feeling like that. My God, how could I ever put this behind me? This is my child too.' When he realized that he should really share his feelings with me our problems disappeared."

PULLING TOGETHER

The death of a baby also has the potential to strengthen a marriage and draw the couple together. Many parents learn a new appreciation for each other through their struggles. When parents communicate their differences and negative feelings, they learn to respond to each other more. Often the couple gain increased respect and admiration for each other. The father expresses appreciation that although the baby died he is grateful that his wife is ok and alive. A mother expresses appreciation for a husband who has been sensitive and who is trying to understand and be patient with her grief.

Many times the marriage becomes the most precious thing the couple has. Though they lost a baby, they still have each other.

"As we look back it seems like it was only a short period that we were on divergent paths. Our marriage is stronger and better than it has ever been. We feel like if we could make it through this we could make it through just about anything."

"One day when we were driving along, out of the blue, my husband started talking about the last year and what we've been through, how far we've come, and the gains that we had made. He said that we should be awfully happy and proud of that. I agreed with him. And then he looked at me and said, 'Especially you. It's been a terrible year for you.' I think that was like lifting something enormous off me. I cried, and I took his hand and said, 'Thank you so much, you couldn't have said anything nicer.' That was a real turning point for us, expressing our gratitude, and his finally understanding what this experience had been like for me."

"At first I wondered about my husband—why wasn't he crying like I was? But I recognized after a year that he deals with death and grief differently than I do. So now I just cry every day, and if Peter cries sometimes or looks like he might cry, I just figure that's the way he deals with it and this is the way I deal with it. I'm not going to think that he doesn't understand me after all this time."

MARRIAGE: DOS AND DON'TS FROM *MOTHERHOOD AND MOURNING*

Larry G. Peppers and Ronald J. Knapp, working extensively with bereaved parents, have made a list to help the mother and father during their bereavement.

MOTHER

1. Grieve in your own way—at your own speed and at your own timing. Recognize that every person is different and unique and you have your own way of grieving.

2. Cry whenever you feel like it and without guilt or wondering about how other people are taking it. Crying is a healthy sign and it is also a necessary part of the grief work. You don't need to apologize.

3. Don't be forced into snap decisions or taking standard treatment because it might be easier. You have a right to weigh the pros and cons of each decision. You have the right to choices and options. You also have the right to take time to make your choices.

4. Try to understand that your husband's grieving is different from yours—not better and not worse—just different. He has been trained by years of culture to hide any expression of grief, and his facade may be very different from the grief he is feeling inside.

FATHER

1. Try to express your feelings. Even though you have been conditioned to hide them, doing so will be destructive to yourself and your marriage. Say what you are feeling when you are feeling it and how you are feeling it. This will open up your marriage and your relationship with your wife.

2. Cry. Show your tears. Try to understand that tears are an important part of the human psyche that have helped relieve the pain of grief and disappointment for millions of years. Don't worry about how others see them and don't apologize for your tears.

3. Establish open communications with your wife by letting her know the depths of your feelings about the baby. It's important for you to try to put yourself in her shoes to recognize the depth of her feelings, her guilt, and her blame for herself. Don't try to hurry her grieving process, you will only prolong it and engender feelings of resentment. Try to recognize the origin of the differences in your feelings. Concentrate on the sameness if you can.

4. If you take time to understand and share things with your wife you will be rewarded tenfold. You may not have learned the skills in the past but any effort will be greatly appreciated.

5. Include your wife in the choices and decision made following the baby's birth and death. Don't be coerced into making all the decisions or make the mistake of thinking that you will be

helping shield her from the pain. Don't let people rush you or her. You have the right to find out about the alternatives and to take the time you need to make the decisions.

6. Try to handle insensitive questions and responses from people around you. Some people don't know what to say or do (you probably didn't either before the death of your baby), and it helps to understand what is behind their inappropriate remarks. Be assertive when handling them, tell people how their remarks make you feel and help them understand your grief. Ignore those people you do not have the energy to deal with.

STRESSES ON SEXUALITY

A major marital area affected by the death may be the couple's sex life. Sex means many things to many people at different times, and at no time more than during grief.

Sex may mean reproduction to the mother: how her baby was conceived, future pregnancies, and even birth. If she enjoys sex it may bring on feelings of guilt. "How could I enjoy myself when my baby is dead?" If she had sex prior to the death of the baby and even subconsciously thinks that it could have caused the miscarriage or premature birth, sex can even be repulsive to her. Sex might mean using a physical and emotional energy that she simply doesn't have.

Sex to the father may mean physical closeness or caring, and it might be the one way he has to show his tenderness and affection. He may think that it shows his wife that she is still attractive to him. On the other hand, he, too, may have feelings of guilt about intercourse as a cause of the baby's death. Or sex to him may mean putting forth a physical and emotional energy that he simply doesn't have, either.

A common scenario is frustration and resentment as the mother, still depressed over the death, cannot think about making love; while the father, thinking that lovemaking shows his affection and concern, may be frustrated by his wife's lack of interest.

Bereaved parents' feelings of anger, guilt, and depression are not conducive to enjoying sex. Problems in communication ending in frustration and resentment suppress sexual desire and the couple's ability to relate sexually. It's hard to express love and affection when feeling physically and emotionally depleted.

The connection between intercourse and the death of their baby creates the fear of conceiving another baby at a time when a woman cannot go through such an experience again. The father also may believe that he couldn't put his wife or himself through such an experience again.

Not all couples experience these feelings about sexuality, however. To some, sexuality is their way of expressing love and comfort. Through lovemaking they are both able to give each other nurturing and comfort.

Many couples want to conceive as soon as they can after the death and as soon as resuming intercourse is appropriate for them. They feel that with their desire to conceive the desire for lovemaking is the best way for them to get over the grief they have just experienced.

It's important for bereaved parents to know that the resumption of intercourse may be difficult for all new parents, and that the lovemaking that accompanies sexual intercourse is more important at this time than the actual act of intercourse. Even parents who have a healthy baby often have problems with sex after the birth. It's important for parents to be patient and gentle, and to allow themselves time to recover. The romantic things they did before marriage are important. A special dinner, a glass of wine, candlelight, a glowing fireplace all help to set up a romantic mood.

AVOIDING SEXUAL DIFFICULTIES DURING BEREAVEMENT

Again, Peppers and Knapp have developed a helpful list of suggestions to help couples avoid and handle many of the sexual difficulties that confront bereaved parents.

1. If you are afraid of a future pregnancy, find and use a

contraceptive that is effective, safe, and easy for you to use. If you find your fears becoming obsessive discuss them with your doctor. You may find that the reasons your baby died have nothing to do with subsequent pregnancies. If the causes are genetic, explore genetic counseling to get a realistic perspective of your fears.

2. Don't let sex become mechanical. Work at keeping the romance in sexuality. Sex is intercourse; sexuality is making love. It is the touch, care, and concern that change a mechanical act into an intimate sexual expression of love.

3. Give yourself time to grieve the death of one child before you try to get pregnant. You cannot replace the baby you lost. Each child must be regarded as unique and individual with his/her own place in the family.

4. Don't allow your loss to lower your self-esteem. You are not alone. Other parents have lost their babies and survived their loss. Other parents in the future will lose their babies. Don't dwell on your failure.

5. Self-denial will not bring your baby back, so don't punish yourself for the death of your baby. Try to participate in the pleasures of life. Take yourself to lunch. Have a new hairdo. Go on a vacation. Splurge on a new outfit—it will do great things for your self-esteem, and you deserve it.

6. Don't worry if you have a decreased sex drive or a lowered libido. These are all normal characteristics of grief and depression. As you work through your grief, your sex drive and libido will return.

7. If you need help don't hesitate to get it. If you feel that your efforts at resuming sex are not moving forward, try sex therapy. It opens up new areas of communication and joy.

SEEKING PROFESSIONAL HELP

Sometimes one parent may be ready to talk about the death while the other hasn't reached that stage yet. It may be that the couple has not developed communication skills in the marriage and doesn't have the ability to help each other. If the relationship is weak, the death may be the breaking point of the marriage. If the relationship is strong, the couple may be able to develop the skills they need.

Understanding the importance of talking and expressing problems and needs can help the couple take definite steps toward discussing the experience. Some parents may be able to do this by themselves, while others need the help of a professional counselor.

Choosing a therapist is the most important decision for parents who have lost their baby and are not able to move through the grief work on their own. It is vital that they find a therapist who has had some previous experience with bereaved parents. Expenses are often a primary concern to a young couple. Many therapists, however, are willing to charge fees on a sliding scale based on ability to pay. Group major medical or other health insurance policies often cover part of the expense. Community health centers usually offer inexpensive or free therapy. Ask your obstetrician or pediatrician for advice in selecting a therapist, or you may want to consult your clergyman.

> "At my three-month follow-up visit, my obstetrician came in and asked me how things were going. I just broke down in tears and, out of nowhere, I said, 'I don't know why Bob doesn't love me anymore.' At that time he suggested we get some counseling. He recommended a psychiatrist who helped me help myself. He helped me learn how to work out of depression and how to understand what Bob was going through."

> "At the time my wife was going through counseling I remember hoping that it would help her. In hoping that it would help her I'd reach out every time she'd

come back and hope there was something that would help me, too. In looking back, I should have gone to counseling too because it was an extremely difficult time for me. I needed help every bit as much as Nancy did."

10

Family, Friends, and Support Groups

FAMILY

Every bereaved parent needs special protection, love, and individual attention. To help parents through the first weeks of grief they need to be surrounded by people who can make them feel good about themselves, who allow the expression of grief, and who will offer emotional support.

Few family members know what to say or even how to articulate their own grief, let alone help and support the bereaved parents.

When told that the pregnancy has ended in death, grandparents and other family may be overwhelmed, and they may have difficulty coping with their own painful emotions. Grandparents may be at a loss for what to say, and rather than say the wrong thing, they say nothing. This may hurt more than anything. Trying to be helpful, family members may indicate that the loss is insignificant. Comments such as, "Well, at least you can have other children," make parents question their own angry thoughts. Some mothers and fathers feel that they have failed the family, failed to produce the healthy grandchild.

Some relatives may appear at the hospital as soon as possible, offering love and understanding.

> "My brother came right away and said there was no way I was staying in the hospital alone. He said they would break down doors to get in. But the hospital was great and let him in. We talked and talked until four-thirty in the morning. He was a great comfort to both me and my husband."

> "I felt that Tom could really use someone near him and so I had his sister come. I felt that helped us both because she took care of the house and all the material things that I needed done. She was close to him and I think that was very nurturing for him."

> "The family was so supportive, until they thought that it was time that I should be bucking up and getting over this thing. It was as if they wanted to push me on."

> "From the very beginning I felt that my friends have been more reliable and available than my own family. I felt so uncomfortable around my parents and especially my sister in discussing it. I wouldn't bring it up and they wouldn't bring it up. So now, I've come to a place where I can discuss it with my mother, but she doesn't discuss it back. We have a barrier that is hard to break down."

GRANDPARENTS: A DOUBLE GRIEF

For grandparents the death of a child is a double blow: the disappointment of their expectations for a grandchild and the pain of seeing their own children suffering. Grandparents share the anticipation of the baby, the excitement of the pregnancy, and the planning of the birth with the parents. They tell their friends about the expected grandchild. Even if they never see the baby, they grieve for its death while wishing they could protect the parents, their children, from their pain.

If the grandmother has also experienced a previous loss, she may wonder secretly if she could be responsible for passing on a problem. Some grandparents suffer survivor guilt. It makes no sense to them that they have survived an infant.

HOW TO HELP

Grandparents who are able to share their feelings play an important part in grief work. Those who are able to cry, to show anger, to be depressed, are better able to provide emotional support. Grandparents who are able to show their grief give the greatest sense of understanding and sharing. When the loss is faced and shared it provides strength to all the family and deepens relationships within the family unit.

Grandparents, however, who conceal their pain in order to provide support are misunderstood by the parents, who view this response as not caring or not understanding. When grandparents ignore or repress their own emotions, the bereaved couple may resent their own parents.

For those parents whose babies survive a few days, the grandparents are able to get to know their grandchildren, and are therefore a great help. They share more love for the baby, and are therefore better able to understand the parents' grief.

The grandparents of those babies with a genetic problem may feel a special guilt, as if they were somehow part of the cause. The feelings of guilt in a family with a history of genetic problems are especially intense.

EXPRESSION OF GRIEF

Grandparents should express their grief openly. In some instances the grandmother may be grieving deeply not only for the baby, but for other losses in her life. Grandparents may find that by allowing the parents to openly discuss the death of the infant their own grief will be worked through.

"When we were driving from Denver to Boulder, my husband kept saying 'My grandson can't be dead. Maybe it was a mistake. Maybe the heartbeat was just weak.' It was a terribly hard thing to accept."

"For weeks after we got home, I could not sleep. All I could think about was my grandchild dead. Nikki and Scott ought to be holding that baby in their arms, and that baby ought to be in that nursery. I had lost my own son before that, and I thought I was going to go crazy after I got home. Finally I came out of it with a strong conviction that we just can't hold on to our children, all we can do is keep on loving them."

"My father gave me a lot of comfort when he told me it's an old Italian belief that when a baby dies, the grandparents who are dead are then receiving and taking care of their grandchild who comes to join them. My baby is even in the same cemetery as my mother's mother and now she has her own three dead little children and my child, too. I told him, 'You know, that is a wonderful thing for me to be able to hold on to.'"

FRIENDS

Friends who want to help ease the pain should realize the parents need to share their anguish and sense of loss. They should understand the need to be able to discuss anger and the sense of failure. The bereaved couple needs to be reassured that their feelings are not crazy, but normal responses to a tragic event.

"Very good friends of ours lost their first and their third child, and their fourth child was brain-damaged. And then they have one son and three daughters that survived, and the two little ones are just supergeniuses. She said, 'We are so sorry to hear of your loss. Our prayers are with you at this time. We know you are going to come through this thing in time, and with a lot of help from your family. We went through this same thing twice, and we know it isn't an easy thing to accept. Right now although little Jimmy (our son who is two) cannot take the place of the little girl you lost, he can help close the place in your heart now that you will always feel for her. Take just one day at a time for a while. We will be thinking of you. God bless.'"

"The most helpful thing my friend did was just to be there when I needed her. There were several times I'd call and say, 'You've got to get down here,' or, 'I'm coming up.' I'm sure it was probably inconvenient at times, but she let me do that. More than any of my friends at that time, she let me talk about my baby and acknowledged his existence. Other friends kept things from me—even their own pregnancies, or they wouldn't talk about Stephan. But never Gail."

"Most of my men friends didn't know what to do or what to say. But I had one friend who would come over and take me for a drive or a game of golf. I remember when everything was very tense and he asked me at one point, 'How do you feel about it?' He wanted to know how I felt. It wasn't like most of the men you talk to. When I would mention anything about the death, they would just say 'fine' and go on to something else—just another piece of business to be dealt with. It helped me tremendously to have somebody who was interested and who cared enough to ask."

"As Nancy's best friend I knew how much she wanted that baby and how devastated she must be by the death. I called Bob and told him that whenever she was ready I would come to see her. At the same time I thought I don't think I can go because I don't know what to say and there's nothing I can do. When Bob finally told me to come over, I spent half an hour trying to get up enough courage to go and see her. When I got there the funny thing was Nancy comforted me. She told me that it was all right to cry. And so we cried together for a while. And then she told me that it was all right not to be able to say anything. And I actually came away feeling better than when I went down. After that I kept in touch with her. I would call her and say 'I don't know what to do. I want to do something for you.' And she would tell me 'Well, this is what I need today!' We were good friends before it happened, but I think it made us a lot closer having gone through it together. We can talk about anything now."

FRIENDS WHO HURT

Some friends say and do things that increase the pain. Especially harmful are those friends who, immediately after the death, act as if nothing had happened at all. This is the most typical response, and the one that is most upsetting. The grief is then compounded by hurt feelings and anger toward those the parents had cared about and counted on most. These friends think they are being helpful by doing nothing, that they are giving time to recuperate.

Other friends, in their attempt to find something positive in the death, leave the parents frustrated. Remarks such as "You will be better parents for having had this experience," or "The baby is with God in heaven," are inappropriate and hard to deal with.

"When I went back to work some of the girls in the office were pregnant. I thought they were very insensitive to my loss when all they talked about was their pregnancies. One day two girls came in and of course they were talking about babies. It was like they were trying to torture me. I couldn't understand. I wanted to go over and stick my scissors through them, but I got up very calmly and went into the restroom, locked myself in the stall, and just almost went hysterical."

"There were a lot of insensitive persons that I felt I had to protect Nancy from. One friend asked the first day when we were planning to have another baby. We just finally had to tell her not to come back."

> "One of my best friends was so disappointing to me because she couldn't seem to let me talk about my baby. She would talk about the weather or her children, but every time we got to me, it was time to go home or time to change the subject. Finally one day she told me, 'I was so afraid that I'd do the wrong thing, and I was so afraid that you didn't want to talk about it that I was always embarrassed when it came up. But I want you to know that anytime you want to talk, I am here.' "

COMMUNICATION DIFFICULTIES: HELPING OTHERS HELP YOU

Friends of bereaved parents want to do the right thing; they want to help, but sometimes they don't know what to do. Here are some guidelines:

1. Friends need to understand the depth of the loss. Parents can tell them: "I never dreamed that it would be so painful." "I need to share my feelings of sadness and grief." "It's so hard because nobody knew this baby, and I feel so alone." "It's important to me to talk about this baby." "The birth, you know, is the only thing that I really feel proud of."

2. Parents often find that everyone wanted to do something for them. Friends are glad of some specific or definite suggestion, if only to do some shopping or help with cooking or cleaning. Most of all the bereaved need time to rest and recuperate, time to be alone. If they have other children they might ask friends for help by giving these children the time and energy the parents don't have. A trip to the zoo or just baby-sitting gives relief. The friends feel better doing something; and in the end, the parents feel better too.

3. Probably one of the most touching experiences is when a family member or a friend (or even a stranger) shares their loss experience. People who have been through grieving have a greater comprehension of the feelings. Such mutual sharing can be encouraged.

4. Many parents find that they develop new friendships with people who had either experienced the death of their own babies, or who are able to share in the grief. These are the people who are able to say the right word or do the right thing at the right moment.

PREGNANT FRIENDS AND FAMILY

Parents may experience a special distance from friends and family who are pregnant themselves. Parents feel a coldness emanating from these people, almost as if their relationship might compromise their success in having a healthy baby. Who wants to be reminded of the possibility of death when pregnant?

> "My sister-in-law was the only one who would listen to me until she became pregnant, and then it was like she couldn't get far enough away from me. Like I had something catching and she and her baby might get it. It was very uncomfortable to be around her."

> "When my sister got pregnant, she told everybody in the family before me. I was so upset. She was my only sister, and we had been very close. I didn't find out until she called and said she needed the information from our genetics counseling. I couldn't understand how my own sister could do this, keep something like this from me."

PARENT SUPPORT GROUPS

Many parents find their greatest solace with other parents who have experienced a similar loss. Parents whose babies have died find that by talking to others (even though they are strangers) they can express their hidden feelings and fears about the death. The nonthreatening and supportive environment helps them to discuss anger, pain, and other emotions and to learn that they are all normal responses to death. This sharing makes support groups an important part of the recovery process. For many it is the only way in which they can begin to recover from the terrible isolation of grief.

"My doctor told me about the parent support group. I didn't wait for them to call me. I called them and talked for a couple of hours. It was the first time that I could talk about it and it didn't make my cry because somebody understood. I talked and even laughed. The mother told me that there was a group meeting and that if I felt like it I should come. I just said, 'Where is it and what time—let me go.'"

"It was reassuring for me to see all the different people—all who had lost their babies. I saw that everyone was laughing and cracking jokes, and it made me feel good to think that I was going to laugh again. Maybe six months from then I could be laughing. And then at the same time, I thought I'm going to be the only one crying and I knew it was okay to cry. It was reassuring to see all these different emotions. And I thought, 'Six months from now I'm going to be okay. I'm going to laugh, and I'm still going to have moments when I cry.' It just gave me a little insight into the future rather than thinking I was going to go crazy."

"I think that it was at a group meeting that I first sat down and listened to a complete account of how my wife felt. We had discussed the death so many times, but never how she felt. I heard some new perspectives on the whole thing, some new things about me and our relationship."

"It was at the group meeting that I learned that my marriage wasn't going to fall apart. People were telling me, 'You're going to grieve differently from your husband. You're going to still be crying and he's going to want to get on with life.' Now that has happened I think it makes it a little easier for me. I'm not surprised when I do cry more than him. I know that I'm normal three months later when I'm still crying and Scott isn't."

11

How to Gather Up the Pieces

REASSESSMENT

Losing a baby forces the parents to reassess everything: religious beliefs, values, their marriage, and their outside relationships. Not only do the parents experience the death of their baby, but they also endure an unexpected loss of dreams for themselves, their families, and their friends. Things can never be as they were before. Bereaved parents can never go back, but they can slowly move forward toward a new growth and a new compassion.

Some parents return to work to try to find needed distractions during the period following the loss; others return to school. Some mothers at home with children throw themselves into the house and children, trying to make some meaning of their lives. Many find that becoming part of a group of parents who have lost their babies gives them great solace. A few parents even start support groups themselves and find that helping other parents with their own experiences gives their babies' deaths some meaning.

LIFE-STYLES

A dramatic change in life-styles may be experienced. The mother may have left her job in expectation of the baby. After the death, she may not be able to get her old position back, or even worse, she may have to face new people in interviews while searching for a job. Many parents don't have the strength or the confidence to meet more challenges, and work may seem meaningless.

SELF-ESTEEM

Self-esteem is at its lowest; parents cannot stand another failure. Anything that contributes to making the parent feel better, no matter how trivial, can be a help in working through grief.

COPING STRATEGIES

Many bereaved parents find that keeping a diary or writing poetry helps give a sense of peace and continuity to the growth experience. Others find that it is essential to face the realization that there are things in life beyond anyone's control.

Some fathers and mothers pamper themselves. Buying new clothes, redecorating the house, joining a health club, or even going on vacation can help to restore some sense of well-being to their lives.

Some couples may find new meaning in their religious affiliations, others devote energy to initiating support groups to help themselves and others.

Having learned how fragile a life can be, parents treasure their other children and their marriages. They appreciate more deeply the love and friendship of those who understood their needs and were there to help.

Most parents plan for future children and discover a stronger commitment toward parenthood than they had ever felt before. They understand how truly miraculous is the life of a breathing, crying, laughing, healthy child.

"If there's anything positive that can come out of a horrible situation like this it is seeing life differently. I think if this had never happened to me, and if I could turn back the clock and I could make it go away, I would, but if this hadn't happened to me I wouldn't have made all these wonderful new friends from our parent support group, and I wouldn't have realized how much a lot of my older friends meant to me. I never realized that they thought so much of me and that they were such wonderful people. I think it opened my eyes to people, and made me see that people are caring and loving, and that there's a lot of good out there."

"I found work really therapeutic. We both went back to work pretty soon and that helped me. All of a sudden it made time go fast. I thought 'I'll never get through that week,' and then it was two weeks ago, and then it was a month ago. I can't say I could recommend work for everybody, but it really helped me."

"We found that the death had changed our lives. Working through our grief helped us to emerge more mature and empathetic to others who have lost a loved one. We are more secure not only in our ability to cope but our ability to survive the other uncertainties of life that are before us."

"The one thing we know now is that death always has been and always will be a part of life. And life is full of uncertainties. It's not like *if* you have problems; it's *when* they are going to happen."

"One thing for sure is that above all, we will never again take children for granted. We appreciate the birth of a healthy baby as one of life's greatest gifts."

III

The Future

12

Subsequent Pregnancies

QUESTIONS THAT HAVE TO BE ANSWERED

After the death of a baby, parents can never again face pregnancy with the same simple innocence. Babies do die. Before parents can consider the responsibility of conceiving, bearing, giving birth to, and possibly losing another baby, some questions must be answered.

- Why did our baby die?
- What are the chances our bodies would betray us again?
- What did the statistics say about our chances now that we have lost one, two, or three babies?
- How long should we wait before we try to conceive again?
- What if we have trouble conceiving again?
- How do we know if we are healed enough to accept another child?
- How do we know if we are healed enough to accept another death?

HOW LONG TO WAIT

Although the question is as individual as the number of couples who ask it, there are general guidelines that may help an interested couple. Parents should let their own feelings be the ultimate guide. Most parents feel they could conceive another child only when they could put behind them the shock, anger, and depression of their grief, when they could be responsible for another unique and individual child. For some this is right after the death of the baby, and for some it takes several years. For others it means pursuing adoption.

There are several factors to be considered before deciding to conceive. These include both the physical and the emotional aspects of recovery.

PHYSICAL RECOVERY

The length of the previous pregnancy, the type of delivery, and the age and health of the mother are all significant factors in determining the time of physical recovery. No woman wants to face another miscarriage after going through the loss of a baby. Most physicians feel that the chances of miscarriage are lessened if the mother allows her body to go through at least three normal menstrual cycles. Some suggest a wait of three to six months after a miscarriage or abortion to give the baby the best physical start possible. If a mother has experienced a stillbirth or infant death, waiting six to twelve months is not uncommon. There are parents who desperately want to conceive again and who must take advantage of every opportunity. Women who feel that their biological clock is running out and who don't have the luxury of waiting six to twelve months, and couples who have had difficulty in conceiving in the first place, have every right to follow their own feelings.

EMOTIONAL RECOVERY

Other factors to be considered are the emotional and psychological recovery of both the mother and the father. Each parent must resolve his/her depression and despair in his/her own time and in his/her own way. Each parent's recovery lies in his/her readiness to accept another child with a separate identity, one who holds its own name and place in the family. If a child is conceived to take the place of the dead baby, that child, the parents, and the other children in the family may suffer long-term effects. The next baby should be loved for him- or herself and should never be compared consciously or unconsciously with the hopes and dreams that the parents had for the baby who died.

Although this may sound cruel and ironic, the parents must have recovered emotionally to have the strength to face another pregnancy, another birth and, as one couple put it, another death, if it is to be.

GENETIC COUNSELING

Some parents may be afraid to become pregnant again due to problems the deceased child had. Most of those who lose a baby, especially for genetic reasons, want to know what the chances are of a repeat experience. Genetic counseling explores the possibilities of the likelihood for future problems.

> "We went to genetic counseling and they couldn't tell us exactly what the problem was, except: 'It could be another problem of recessive genes. If that's the case you have a twenty-five percent chance of it happening again. Those are your odds and that's about all we can tell you.' That was a blow because all of a sudden we were in limbo, we didn't know where we stood. Not knowing was very difficult for me."

"When we finally did decide to have another baby, we went to a specialist to be sure this baby wouldn't be born with the same chromosomal abnormality as Stephan. After amniocentesis and ultrasound we were supremely relieved that we were carrying a 'normal' baby. But, emotionally, we didn't believe it until she was born alive and well."

THE DECISION

The decision to conceive another baby is easier for some parents than for others. There are parents who decide to have another baby as soon as possible. Other parents need time to work through the grief, and don't have the strength or energy to consider conception for a while. As the pain dulls and life resumes, they may find the desire and courage to plan another pregnancy.

It seems to be more common for the father to be ready for another pregnancy before the mother is. These couples need time and patience, and perhaps special counseling to help bring them together.

Parents who have experienced multiple losses must face the tragic possibility that they may never conceive and give birth to a healthy baby. Although some options have been closed down, there are still others open. These parents could choose to face the fact that they would never have a family and fill their lives with other creative endeavors such as teaching, helping with children's groups, writing, art, or work. Or they could choose the route of adoption. Those who do adopt are then faced with a wholly new and difficult journey.

"I think most doctors say: 'You can get pregnant in three months.' I think they should preface that with 'Wait three months and then you can start thinking about trying to get pregnant again. And don't be alarmed at all if it takes six months or a year.' I think I was really lucky to get pregnant as quickly as I did, but I would have been very apprehensive had I not."

"We weren't getting any younger, and as we had some problem conceiving in the first place, we decided to go ahead and have another baby as fast as we could. For us, it was just right. The baby, born a year after our other one, has brought us the greatest happiness we ever thought possible. He filled our life and made us a complete family. Of course I miss our other baby, but it only makes me appreciate our son that much more."

"I just couldn't think about having another baby now. It takes every bit of strength I have just to get out of bed—how could I think about parenting a new baby? Or worse yet, how could I think about losing another baby? I know my husband is ready, but I'm not."

"I thought I could never consider having another baby. But after a year of grieving and crying, I find I am beginning to laugh and enjoy life again, and beginning to think that life without another baby would be the real tragedy. And I'm happy to say that we are pregnant again, and looking forward to this baby."

"It was really a sore point in our marriage. I wanted to get on with having a family. Neither of us was getting any younger. And all my wife did was cry and grieve and mourn. It was a tough time."

ONCE THE DECISION IS MADE: A TIME FOR FEARS

Although the decision to conceive another child may have solved one question, it only opens up a whole new set of fears that need to be faced and resolved.

"I couldn't go through another pregnancy with my doctor saying, 'Don't worry. Everything will be just fine. You are just fine. Your blood pressure is wonderful!' I had been through that before and my baby died at birth. Fortunately, when I went in the doctor said to me, 'This pregnancy is going to be really rough. You have been through a terrible ordeal, and you are going to need a lot of support.' I don't know what books he has read, or who he talked to between the death of my baby and this time, but he said the right thing to me—the only thing that could give me reassurance."

"I was really concerned from the beginning that my doctor was going to pat my shoulder and tell me not to worry. I was so relieved when I asked him, 'What if this happens again?' He said, 'Well, I'll tell you, Ardee, if this happens again, you're going to have to pick up the pieces and start all over—and that's just the way it's going to be.' I said, 'I'm really glad you said that because you are being honest with me and you are right.' "

FEAR OF CONCEPTION

For some it was difficult to conceive in the first place. It will be doubly difficult to try again. Mothers in their thirties have special fears of not being able to succeed. Each menstrual period is a sign of the failure and inability to do even the most elemental of all functions.

> "After we made the decision, we thought that we would just miraculously get pregnant right away. Well, that didn't happen. Month after month my first sign of menstruation would throw me into great depression. This went on for a year. We went in for fertility tests and put ourselves through all sorts of junk. Then, just as I had given up and went in for a regular checkup the doctor told me I was pregnant. Just like that my world turned around."

> "The only anxiety I have about being pregnant again is, 'Is it ever going to happen?' I was amazed the first time that I got pregnant. But I've resigned myself that it's probably going to take a long time. I realize that it could be a month from now, or it could be a year or two years. Well, it's just something I'm going to have to learn to live with."

FEAR OF MISCARRIAGE

Once conception has occurred, parents must go through the torment of fearing with each sign that their bodies might fail them. This anguish continues until they pass the time when they had lost the other baby. Even then, it is difficult to enjoy the new pregnancy.

"There wasn't a gas pain or a sneeze that didn't become a signal to me of another miscarriage. When I became pregnant with this baby I didn't allow myself a glass of wine or cup of coffee. I became Mrs. Good Girl. There was nothing I wouldn't do to keep this baby."

"I wondered what happened. Here I was supposed to be so happy and joyful. And my pregnancy was just like gloom and doom, until I passed my first trimester when I had lost the other baby. And then I just knew my baby was going to make it, and then I started to cheer up."

FEAR OF CARRYING AN UNVIABLE BABY

Some parents need to know what the chances are for this baby to survive. They undergo batteries of tests to determine if the child is going to be healthy and normal.

Between the 15th and 17th week of gestation there are several procedures that may be used to help determine the condition of the fetus. Not until the results of these tests are reported can parents begin to believe that they have a chance for a normal, healthy baby. The waiting period is excruciating.

"I remember waiting for the amniocentesis results to come back. It seemed like a good part of our life was spent waiting. First we waited for the chromosome test. Then we waited for the genetic counseling. We waited for autopsy reports that came four months later. Then we waited to get pregnant. Only to wait for the sixteenth week to get the amniocentesis results. When we finally got the results that told us our daughter seemed to be perfect in every way we began to wait for the birth. But at least we could begin to relax a little."

FEAR DURING PREGNANCY

Throughout the whole pregnancy, the mother is searching for signs of a healthy baby. She may worry if the baby has moved too much or not enough. Through the pregnancy she may be overly conscientious of her health. Some may become obsessive about their weight gains. If a mother catches a cold or the flu she may be concerned how this will affect her baby.

> "With my first pregnancy, I knew I was pregnant and I was going to have a healthy baby. I just took it for granted and really didn't think about it. I never thought twice about death before. I never thought, during my life, that my baby would die. Now that I am pregnant with this baby I think about it constantly. I find myself *willing* this baby to be born alive."

> "When the first baby was conceived it was like, 'Great, wonderful!' This time all the way through it was like I couldn't be happy about it. I couldn't plan. I couldn't do anything."

> "It's really funny. This time everybody is cautious. Our family and friends. It's like they are afraid to get too involved. They are afraid that, 'Oh, my God, if something happens again, we're going to have to go through all this again.'"

FEAR OF CHILDBIRTH

Parents who went through labor and delivered a stillborn child can never shake the fear that the next baby will not be delivered alive, safe, and healthy. Not until the baby is placed in their arms and has survived through the first days of life can they allow themselves to begin to accept the fact that they can and did deliver a healthy baby.

"I went into labor two weeks early and just knew that the baby couldn't survive. After all our practicing and Lamaze classes I just went to pieces. My husband kept telling me to breathe and relax. He tried so hard and I wouldn't do anything he said. Our son was born seven and a half pounds of healthy boy—and of course I was happy, but I couldn't get over being disappointed that the birth was early, I wasn't prepared, and I did so poorly."

FEAR DURING POSTPARTUM

During the few days following birth of a healthy baby, parents may grieve for their earlier lost baby. They compare the live, healthy baby with the dead one: the similarities and differences between the pregnancies, the childbirth experience, and the possible personalities of the children. Some parents find that it takes time to become secure and comfortable that this new baby will not die too.

It is not unusual for parents to question their doctor and nurse constantly. The parents may see problems in the new baby that do not exist, but having lost one they are concerned that the new baby may die also.

"I expected feelings of motherhood to descend over me like a curtain. I was disappointed when I felt a sort of numbness. I wondered what was wrong with me. It wasn't until they brought the baby to me, let me feed and dress her, that I began to feel that maybe she would make it. I wished someone would have prepared me for these feelings because I really felt guilty."

"The first part was like a dream. I couldn't believe it was all happening. It really took me a couple of days to attach to my new baby. After that they couldn't get her out of my arms. I didn't trust anyone with her and I didn't want her out of my sight."

AT HOME

Once the new baby is home, parents encounter new problems. Although they know the baby is OK, parents may feel ambivalent toward the child as they resolve, once again, grief for the dead child. There may be a tendency to make this the perfect baby and the perfect experience. But as they contend with colic, diaper rash, and spit ups, resentment because their fantasies and expectations are unrealistic begins to build. After all, it seems as if they deserve the perfect baby. The realities of parenthood can be overwhelming for the couple.

"Two years and two months after Stephan's death, we had a second child. We had gone through the amniocentesis and we had been told that he was fine, but it didn't stop the worrying. And not until he was delivered and I heard his cry did I know that he was all right, and I felt relieved. When we got home with Timothy, we spent the whole day grieving for Stephan because we saw what we had missed."

"I kept trying to act happy and excited because I knew that everyone expected me to. But I was really experiencing deep feelings of sorrow for my baby who had died. I spent hours thinking how different it would have been if our first baby had survived."

Epilogue

Since we first conceived and gave birth to our book *Death of a Dream,* each couple's life has changed considerably. Some went on to have other children, one is divorced, several are still trying, and one adopted children. Life goes on. The pain never goes away entirely, but it does subside and take on new dimensions. None of the parents will ever be the same, or look on pregnancy and birth in the same way they did before they suffered their loss.

JUDY and STEVEN (Miscarriage–6 weeks)
Sherry–11 months

CINDY and ALLEN (Miscarriage–16 weeks)
Divorced

LOIS and JOHN (Multiple Miscarriages)
Mary–3 years (adopted)
Tommy–4 years (adopted)

CHRISTY and JAMES (Stillbirth–38 weeks)
Pamela–15 months

KATHERINE and LARRY (Stillbirth–40 weeks)
Alexander–9 months

JANET and PAUL (Newborn Death)
Jimmy–6 years
Jonathan–21 months

RHONDA and HARRY (Newborn Death)
Timothy–4½ years
Megan–15 months

SANDY and CHARLES (Early Infant Death)
No children

Appendix

Support Groups for Bereaved Parents

THE SOCIETY OF COMPASSIONATE FRIENDS
(over 270 branches throughout the U.S.)

International Headquarters:
109 Lillington Road
Leamington Spa
Warwickshire
England CV32 6LJ

U.S. Headquarters:
P.O. Box 1347
Oak Brook, IL 60521

CALIFORNIA

S.A.N.D.
c/o Janet Kirksey
Alta Bates Hospital
Berkeley, CA 94705

A.M.E.N.D.
4032 Towhee Drive
Calabassas, CA 91302

R.E.S.P.O.N.D.
c/o Kathy Sorrels
10 Forest Creek Circle
Chico, CA 95926

S.H.A.R.E.
c/o Diana Brenseth
5854 East Lansing
Fresno, CA 93727

H.A.N.D.
c/o Ginger Valen
19 West Gate Way
San Anselmo, CA 94960

COLORADO

BOULDER COUNTY STILLBORN/NEWBORN LOSS SUPPORT GROUP
c/o Marcia Lattanzi
Boulder County Hospice
Boulder, CO 80302

ROSE MEDICAL CENTER
c/o Mary Krugman, Coordinator
Parent Education Program
4567 East Ninth Avenue
Denver, CO 80220

CONNECTICUT

BEREAVED PARENTS
c/o Nancy Baranowski
28 Wesley Drive
Huntington, CT 06484

FLORIDA

H.O.P.E.S. (Helping Other Parents Experience Sorrow)
c/o Sandi Poston
P. O. Box 1143
Lutz, FL 33549

A.M.E.N.D.
c/o Dottie Cannon
5104 127th Avenue
Tampa, FL 33617

ILLINOIS

A.M.E.N.D.
c/o Jane Borman
2209 Gillis
Alton, IL 62002

S.H.A.R.E.
c/o Cecilia Ringhoeffer
St. Elizabeth's Hospital
Pastoral Care Department
211 South Third Street
Belleville, IL 62221
(618-234-2120)

S.H.A.R.E.
c/o Claudia and Tony Klesert
St. Anthony's Memorial Hospital
Auxiliary Room
Carbondale, IL 62901
(618-549-3007)

S.H.A.R.E.
Memorial Hospital of Carbondale
404 West Main Street
Carbondale, IL 62901

S.H.A.R.E.
c/o Marilyn James
Effingham, IL 62401
(217-683-2210)

S.H.A.R.E.
St. Anthony Hospital
503 Maple Street
Effingham, IL 62401

S.H.A.R.E.
c/o Sharon and Terry Maggart
853 West College Street
Jacksonville, IL 62650
(217-245-7668)

S.H.A.R.E.
Passavant Area Hospital
1600 West Walnut Street
Jacksonville, IL 62650

S.H.A.R.E.
St. Francis Hospital
1215 East Union
Litchfield, IL 62056

S.H.A.R.E.
c/o Gregory and Joanne Matzke
10301 Medill
Melrose Park, IL 60164
(Chicago area)

COMPASSIONATE FRIENDS (for parents who've lost older children)
P. O. Box 1347
Oak Brook, IL 60521
(They publish a newsletter, subscription $5.00 a year.)

P.A.C.E.S. (Parent and Child Education Society)
Bereaved Parents
c/o Cathy McMeilly
619 South Humphrey
Oak Park, IL 60304

S.H.A.R.E.
St. Francis Hospital Medical Center
530 N.E. Glen Oak
Peoria, IL 61637

S.H.A.R.E.
Blessing Hospital
10005 Broadway
Quincy, IL 62301

S.H.A.R.E.
St. Mary's Hospital
1415 Vermont
Quincy, IL 62301

S.H.A.R.E.
Rockford Memorial Hospital
2400 North Rockton
Rockford, IL 61103

S.H.A.R.E.
c/o Sister Jane Marie Lamb
St. John's Hospital
800 East Carpenter
Springfield, IL 62702
(217-544-6464, ext. 4500)
(They publish a newsletter, free.)

S.H.A.R.E.
c/o Sandra D. Dunn
Mercy Hospital
1400 West Park
Urbana, IL 61801

INDIANA

BEREAVED PARENTS GROUP
Parents and Friends of Children
c/o Linda Runden
622 North Capitol Avenue
Corydon, IN 47112

PROJECT COMFORT
c/o Gerald C. Machgan, Chaplain
Parkview Hospital
2200 Randalia Drive
Fort Wayne, IN 46805

NEO FIGHT
c/o Pam Dickerson
4815 North Kenyon Drive
Indianapolis, IN 46226

IOWA

EMPTY ARMS
c/o Dr. Russell Striffler
St. Luke's Methodist Hospital
1026 A. Avenue, N.E.
Cedar Rapids, IA 52402

KANSAS

BEREAVED PARENTS OF PITTSBURG
c/o Mrs. Howard Thompson
Quincy & Bypass
Pittsburg, KS 66762

KENTUCKY

NORTON CHILDREN'S HOSPITAL
c/o Chaplain Wayne Willis
P. O. Box 35070
Louisville, KY 40232

MASSACHUSETTS

BOSTON HOSPITAL FOR WOMEN
c/o Anne Groves, Director
Social Services
221 Longwood Avenue
Boston, MA 02115

C.O.P.E.
37 Clarendon Street
Boston, MA 02116

H.O.P.E.
c/o Susan Harrington
South Shore Hospital
55 Fogg Road
South Weymouth, MA 02190

BOSTON STILLBIRTH STUDY GROUP
c/o Ann Ross, Jean Stringham, and Judith Riley
53 Country Corners Road
Wayland, MA 01778

GRIEF SUPPORT GROUP
Childbirth Education Association of Central Massachusetts
c/o Linda Brink and Merilyn Bambauer
P. O. Box 193, West Side Station
Worcester, MA 01602

MICHIGAN

P.E.N.D. (Parents Experiencing Neonatal Death)
c/o Neonatal I.C.U. Marcia Eager
Butterworth Hospital
Grand Rapids, MI 49503

SURVIVORS UP FROM GRIEF
17125 Fordline
Riverview, MI 48192

BEREAVED PARENTS GROUP
c/o Betty Rabant
St. Bede's Church
18290 West Twelve Mile Road
Southfield, MI 48076

MINNESOTA

PARENTS' GRIEF SUPPORT GROUP
c/o Judy Zehren
Route 1 Box 20006
Britts, MN 55710

PARENTS' GRIEF SUPPORT GROUP
c/o Kathy Peterson
St. Mary's Hospital
Duluth, MN 55805

MISSOURI

PARENTS IN CRISIS
c/o Sue Hiesten
303 Brewer
Columbia, MO 65201

MOTHERS IN CRISIS
c/o Terry Weston
Social Services Department
Freeman Hospital
Joplin, MO 64801

A.M.E.N.D.
c/o Maureen Connelly
4324 Berrywick
St. Louis, MO 63128

NEW JERSEY

HELP (for parents who've lost babies or children)
c/o Eileen Thompson
Ventnor, NJ 08406
(609-822-5265)

NEW YORK

BEREAVEMENT CLINIC
c/o Joanne Middleton
Downstate Medical Center
450 Clarkson Avenue
Brooklyn, NY 11203

S.H.A.R.E.
c/o Lois Sugarman
6726 Gleason Place
Fayetteville, NY 13066

MISCARRIAGE AND STILLBIRTH SUPPORT GROUP
c/o Dorothy Hai
209 York Street
Olean, NY 14760

NORTH CAROLINA

PARENT CARE, INC.
c/o Lil Galphin
Box 125
Cary, NC 27511

KINDER-MOURN, INC.
605 East Boulevard
Charlotte, NC 28203

OHIO

BEREAVED PARENTS GROUP
3136 Ellet Avenue
Akron, OH 44312

S.H.A.R.E.
c/o Marilyn Miller Graef
1272 Indian Hill Drive
Bolivar, OH 44612

P.E.N.D.
Rainbow Babies and Children's Hospital
2101 Adelbert Road
Cleveland, OH 44106

PARENT SUPPORT GROUP
Childbirth Education Association of Akron
c/o Linda Baily
2183 Larchdale
Guy Falls, OH 44221

OKLAHOMA

A.M.E.N.D.
1344 East 26th Place
Tulsa, OK 74100

PENNSYLVANIA

S.H.A.R.E.
P. O. Box 961
Lancaster, PA 17604

BOOTH MATERNITY HOSPITAL GRIEF PROCESS GROUP
c/o Dr. Nancy Johns and Laurie Rendall
6051 Overbrook Avenue
Philadelphia, PA 19131

GRIEVING CLINIC
c/o Dr. Susan Jasin
Temple University Health Sciences Center
3401 North Broad Street
Philadelphia, PA 19140

U.N.I.T.E.
Jeans Hospital
7600 Central Avenue
Philadelphia, PA 19111

TENNESSEE

P.E.N.D.
P. O. Box 38445
Germantown, TN 38138

TEXAS

H.O.P.E.
c/o Karen Riley, R.N.
14207 Locke Lane
Houston, TX 77077

S.H.A.R.E. OF SAN ANTONIO
The Harbor
3534 Avenue B
San Antonio, TX 78209

UTAH

SHARING HEART
c/o Thomas D. Coleman
University of Utah Medical Center
Department of Pediatrics, Room 2B425
50 North Medical Drive
Salt Lake City, UT 84132

WASHINGTON

P.E.N.D.
c/o Laurie Lowen
13613 N.E. 26th Place
Bellevue, WA 98005

PARENTS OF STILLBORNS
Group Health Cooperative East Side
Redmond, WA 98052

PARENTS OF STILLBORNS
c/o Bill and Doreen Dolleman
6210 South 120th Street
Seattle, WA 98178

WISCONSIN

S.H.A.R.E.
St. Vincent Hospital
P. O. Box 1220
Green Bay, WI 54305

S.H.A.R.E.
St. Francis Medical Center
700 West Avenue South
LaCrosse, WI 54601

S.H.A.R.E.
Lutheran Hospital
1910 South Avenue
LaCrosse, WI 54601

BEREAVED PARENTS SUPPORT GROUP
c/o Carol Fowler
1016 Van Buren Street
Madison, WI 53711
(608-257-6352)

A.I.I.D. (Aid In Infant Death)
Childbirth Education Association
5636 West Burleigh
Milwaukee, WI 53210

S.H.A.R.E.
St. Nicholas Hospital
2419 Saemann Avenue
Sheboygan, WI 53081

PARENTS SUPPORTING PARENTS
c/o Mary Berg, R.N.
Rice Clinic
2501 Main Street
Stevens Point, WI 54481

Bibliography

WORKS CITED

Apgar, Virginia, and Beck, Joan. *Is My Baby All Right?* New York: Trident, 1973.

Arnstein, Helene S. *What to Tell Your Child: About Birth, Illness, Death, Divorce, and Other Family Crises.* rev. ed. Westport, Conn.: Condor Publishing, 1978.

Benedek, Therese. "The Psychobiology of Pregnancy." In *Parenthood: Its Psychology and Psychopathology,* edited by James Anthony and Therese Benedek. Boston: Little, Brown, 1970.

Benfield, D. Gary, Leib, Susan A., and Vollman, John H. "Grief Response of Parents to Neonatal Death and Parent Participation in Deciding Care." *Pediatrics* 62:2 (August 1978).

Bereavement and Marriage Stress. Commack, N.Y.: Compassionate Friends, 1978.

Bibring, Grete L. "Some Considerations of the Psychological Processes in Pregnancy." *Psychoanalytic Study of the Child.* vol. 14. New York: International University Press, 1959.

Boston Women's Health Book Collective. *Our Bodies, Ourselves.* 2d ed. New York: Simon & Schuster, 1976.

Bowlby, John. *Attachment and Loss.* New York: Basic Books, 1969.

Brazelton, T. Berry. "When a Baby Is Born Too Early." *Redbook* 154, no. 1 (November 1979), pp. 53, 119–121.

Cain, Albert, and Cain, Barbara. "On Replacing a Child." *Journal of American Academy of Child Psychiatry* 3 (1964), pp. 443–455.

———, Fast, I., and Erickson, M. E. "Children Disturbed by the Death of a Sibling." *American Journal of Orthopsychiatry* 34 (1964).

Caplan, Gerald, M.D. "The Mental Hygiene Role of the Nurse in Maternal and Child Care." *Nursing Outlook* 1954, Boston University School of Nursing (August 1968).

———. "Patterns of Parental Response to the Crisis of Premature Birth: A Preliminary Approach to Modifying the Mental Health Outcome." *Psychiatry* 23 (1960), pp. 365–374.

———. "Practical Steps for the Family Physician in the Prevention of Emotional Disorders." *Journal of the American Medical Association* (July 1959), pp. 1497–1506.

———. *Principles of Preventive Psychiatry.* New York: Basic Books, 1964.

Chase, Helen C. "Perinatal Mortality: Overview and Current Trends." *Clinics in Perinatology* 1:1 (March 1974).

Clayton, Paula, M.D., et al. "A Study of Normal Bereavement." *American Journal of Psychiatry* 125 (August 2, 1968), pp. 64–74.

Colman, Arthur D., and Colman, Libby L. *Pregnancy: The Psychological Experience.* New York: The Seabury Press, 1972.

Cullberg, J. "Mental Reactions of Women to Perinatal Death." *Psychosomatic Medicine in Obstetrics and Gynaecology,* 3rd International Congress, London 1971. Basel: S. Karger AG, 1972.

Dunlop, Joyce. "Bereavement Reaction Following Stillbirth." *The Practitioner* 222 (1979), pp. 45–51.

Elia, Andrew D. "The Management of Grief Situations in Obstetrics." *The Boston Medical Quarterly* 10:1 (March 1959).

Engel. "Grief and Grieving." *American Journal of Nursing* 64:9 (September 1964), pp. 93–98.

Fulton, Robert. "On the Dying of Death." In *Explaining Death to Children,* edited by Earl A. Grollman. Boston: Beacon Press, 1967.

Furman, Erna P. "The Death of a Newborn: Care of the Parents." *Birth and the Family Journal* 5:4 (Winter 1978).

Giles, P. F. H. "Reactions of Women to Perinatal Death." *Australian and New Zealand Journal of Obstetrics and Gynecology* 10:207 (1970).

Guttmacher, Alan F. *Pregnancy, Birth, and Family Planning.* New York: Signet, 1973.

Hardgrove, Carol, and Warrick, Louise H. "Perinatal Death: The

Grieving Mother." *American Journal of Nursing* 74:3 (March 1974).

Jensen, Joseph, and Zahouvek, Roslyn. "Depression in Mothers Who Have Lost a New Born." *Rocky Mountain Medical Journal* (November 1972).

Kaplan, David, and Mason, Edward A. "Maternal Reactions to Premature Birth Viewed as an Acute Emotional Disorder." *American Journal of Orthopsychiatry* 30:3 (July 1960), pp. 539–552.

Kaplan, Louise J. *Oneness and Separateness: From Infant to Individual.* New York: Simon & Schuster, 1978.

Kennell, John H., M.D., et al. "The Mourning Response of Parents to the Death of a Newborn Infant." *New England Journal of Medicine* 283 (August 1970), pp. 344–349.

Klaus, Marshall H., and Kennell, John H. *Maternal-Infant Bonding.* St. Louis: C. V. Mosby, 1976.

Kowalski, K., and Bowes, W. "Parents' Response to a Stillborn Baby." *Contemporary Obstetrics and Gynecology* 8 (October 1976), pp. 53–57.

Kübler-Ross, Elisabeth. *On Death and Dying.* New York: The Macmillan Company, 1969.

Lee, Kwang-Sun, Paneth, Nigel, Gartner, Lawrence M., Pearlman, Mark A., and Gruss, Leslie. "Neonatal Mortality: An Analysis of the Recent Improvement in the United States." *American Journal of Public Health* 70, no. 1 (January 1980), pp. 15–21.

Lieberman, James. "Preventive Psychiatry and Family Planning." *Journal of Marriage and the Family* (November 1964), pp. 471–477.

Lewis, Emanuel. "The Management of Stillbirth: Coping with an Unreality." *The Lancet* (September 18, 1976).

———. "Mourning by the Family After a Stillbirth or Neonatal Death." *Archives of Diseases of Childhood* 54 (1979).

———. "Reactions to Stillbirth." *Proceedings of the Third International Congress of Psychosomatic Medicine in Obstetrics and Gynaecology.* Basel: S. Karger AG, 1972, pp. 323–325.

———, and Page, Anne. "Failure to Mourn a Stillbirth: An Overlooked Catastrophe." *British Journal of Medical Psychology* 51 (1978), pp. 237–241.

Lewis, Thomas H. "A Culturally Patterned Depression in a Mother After Loss of a Child." *Psychiatry* 38 (February 1975), pp. 92–95.

Lifton, Robert J. "Advocacy and Corruption in the Healing Professions." In *Nourishing the Humanistic in Medicine,* edited by William R. Rogers and David Barnard. Pittsburgh: University of Pittsburgh Press, 1979, pp. 53–72.

Lindemann, Erich. "Symptomatology and Management of Acute Grief." *American Journal of Psychiatry* 101 (1944), pp. 141–148.

Malmquist, A., Kaij, L., and Nilsson, A. "Psychiatric Aspects of Spontaneous Abortion. I. A Matched Control Study of Women with Living Children." *Journal of Psychosomatic Research* 13 (1969), pp. 45–51.

Mann, Edward. "Spontaneous Abortions and Miscarriages." *Modern Perspectives in Psycho-obstetrics.* Edited by John G. Howell. New York: Brunner/Mazel, 1972.

Miles, Margaret Shandor. "The Grief of Parents . . . When a Child Dies." Mimeograph published by The Compassionate Friends, Oak Brook, Illinois, 1980.

Newton, Michael. "Other Complications of Labor." In *Obstetrics and Gynaecology,* edited by David L. Danforth. 3rd ed. New York: Harper & Row, 1977.

Parkes, Colin Murray. "Bereavement and Mental Illness, Part 2. A Classification of Bereavement Reactions." *British Journal of Medical Psychology* 38 (1965), pp. 13–26.

———. *Bereavement: Studies of Grief in Adult Life.* New York: International Universities Press, 1972.

———. "The Nature of Grief." *International Journal of Psychiatry* (1967), pp. 435–438.

Pizer, Hank, and Palinski, Christine O'Brien. *Coping with a Miscarriage.* New York: Dial, 1980.

Pritchard, Jack A., and MacDonald, Paul C., eds. *Williams Obstetrics.* 16th ed. New York: Appleton-Century-Crofts, 1980.

Schiff, Harriet Sarnoff. *The Bereaved Parent.* Harmondsworth, Middlesex: Penguin Books, 1977.

Seitz, Pauline M., and Warrick, Louise H. "Perinatal Death: The Grieving Mother." *American Journal of Nursing* 74:11 (November 1974).

Thaler, Otto F. "Grief and Depression." *Nursing Forum* 5, no. 2 (1966), pp. 9–22.

Ujhely, Gertrude B. "Grief and Depression: Implications for Preventive and Therapeutic Nursing Care." *Nursing Forum* 5, no. 2 (1966), pp. 23–35.

U.S., Department of Health, Education and Welfare. *Public Health Service: Antenatal Diagnosis.* Washington, D.C.: National Institutes of Health Publication (April 1979).

U.S., Department of Health, Education and Welfare. *Healthy People: The Surgeon General's Report on Health Promotion and Disease Prevention.* Pub. no. 79-55071. Washington, D.C.: Government Printing Office (1979).

U.S., Department of Health and Human Services. *Vital and Health Statistics.* Hyattsville, Md: National Center of Health Statistics. Monthly publications.

Volkan, Vamik. "Typical Findings in Pathological Grief." *Psychiatric Quarterly* (April 1970), pp. 1–20.

Wolff, John R., Nielson, Paul E., and Schiller, Patricia. "The Emotional Reaction to a Stillbirth." *American Journal of Obstetrics and Gynecology* 108:1 (September 1, 1970), pp. 73–77.

FURTHER READING

Berezin, Nancy. *After a Loss in Pregnancy.* New York: Simon & Schuster, A Fireside Book, 1982. Help for families affected by a miscarriage, a stillbirth or the loss of a newborn. The special forces that work for and against the recovery of bereaved mothers.

Borg, Susan, and Lasker, Judith. *When Pregnancy Fails.* Boston; Beacon Press, 1981. Families coping with miscarriage, stillbirth, and infant death, and the networks that support them.

Friedman, Rochelle, M.D., and Gradstein, Bonnie, M.P.H. *Surviving Pregnancy Loss.* Boston: Little, Brown, 1981. Describes relations of/reactions to pregnancy loss and practical approaches to coping with emotional problems.

Jimenz, Sherry L. *The Other Side of Pregnancy: Coping with Miscarriage and Stillbirth.* Englewood Cliffs, N.J.: Prentice-Hall Inc., 1982. For parents and health professionals.

Kübler-Ross, Elisabeth. *Questions and Answers on Death and Dying.* New York: Macmillan Publishing Co., 1974. Pioneer work on what the dying have to teach doctors, nurses, clergy, and their own families. Classic work on stages of grieving.

Klaus, Marshall, and Kennel, John. *Maternal-Infant Bonding: The Impact of Early Separation or Loss on Family Development.* Canada: C. V. Mosby Co. Ltd., 1976. Written for professionals dealing with parents whose babies are ill, deformed, or dying.

Knapp, Ronald, and Peppers, Larry. *Motherhood and Mourning: Perinatal Death.* New York: Praeger Publishers, 1980. Information on the effects of fetal/infant death on mothers, covering stages of grief and marital conflicts, doctor-patient relations, communications in hospital.

Kushner, Harold. *When Bad Things Happen to Good People.* New York: Avon Books, 1983. Inspirational book covering response to loss and grief.

Schiff, Harriet S. *The Bereaved Parent.* New York: Penguin Books, 1978. Book covers daily decisions and hardships confronting parents whose child has died.

Index